WIRED FOR SOUND

An Advanced Student Workbook on Hearing and Hearing Aids

written by

Carole Bugosh Simko

illustrated by

Jan Skrobisz

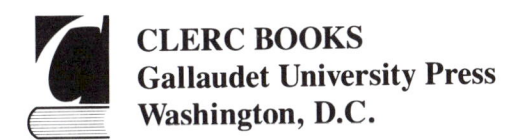

CLERC BOOKS
Gallaudet University Press
Washington, D.C.

Clerc Books
An imprint of Gallaudet University Press
Washington, DC 20002
© 1986 by Gallaudet University. All rights reserved
Published 1986
Second printing, 1990
Printed in the United States of America

ISBN 0-930323-16-5

Cover design by Jan Skrobisz

Dedicated to my husband
and my parents

CONTENTS

Why You Should Read This Book — 1

PART I *All About Hearing*

LESSON 1	*How We Hear*	5
LESSON 2	*Different Kinds of Hearing Loss*	12
LESSON 3	*How Hearing Is Tested*	21
LESSON 4	*Understanding Your Audiogram*	28
LESSON 5	*Questions About Your Hearing*	36
LESSON 6	*How Do You Feel About Your Hearing Loss?*	43

PART II *All About Hearing Aids*

LESSON 7	*How a Hearing Aid Helps You*	53
LESSON 8	*Hearing Aids*	56
LESSON 9	*Hearing Aid Check*	69
LESSON 10	*Important Hearing Aid Information*	71
LESSON 11	*Questions People Ask About Hearing Aids*	76
LESSON 12	*What a Hearing Aid Can and Cannot Do*	82
LESSON 13	*When Could You Have Trouble Hearing?*	84
LESSON 14	*What Can You Do to Hear Better?*	86
LESSON 15	*How Do You Feel About Your Hearing Aid?*	88
LESSON 16	*Hearing Aid Care*	96
LESSON 17	*Hearing Aid Parts*	105
LESSON 18	*Fixing Hearing Aid Problems*	133

Summary — 139
Answer Key — 140

Why You Should Read This Book

You are a very special person because you wear a hearing aid. Only special people wear hearing aids.

You probably have special questions about your hearing and hearing aid. Have you ever wondered why you have a hearing problem? Will your hearing ever get better? How does an aid help you to hear better? When should you wear the aid? Which kind of hearing aid do you wear? Do you know how to take good care of the aid? Can you fix small problems with it? How do you feel about having a hearing loss? How do you feel about wearing an aid?

All of your questions are important. Each question should be answered. This book will help you to answer those questions. It will help you to answer many other questions, too.

PART I

All About Hearing

Lesson 1

How We Hear

New Vocabulary

You will learn these words as you read this lesson. Say each word. Read its definition.

Cochlea: a part of the inner ear. It is shaped like a snail. There are many tiny nerve endings inside the cochlea.

Decibel: a unit for measuring how loud or soft a sound is.

Ear: the part of the body that helps us hear. The ear is divided into three main sections.

Ear canal: the passage that carries sound from the pinna to the eardrum.

Eardrum: a small opening inside the ear that is covered with skin. The eardrum moves back and forth when sound hits it. The eardrum lies between the outer ear and the middle ear.

Frequency: the number of sound waves per second a sound makes. The frequency tells how high or low a sound is.

Hammer, anvil, and stirrup: the three tiny bones in the middle ear. These are the smallest bones in the body.

Hearing nerve: a nerve that stretches from the cochlea to the brain. It carries messages from the ear to the brain.

Hertz: a unit for measuring the frequency of a sound.

Inner ear: the third section of the ear. We cannot see it. It contains the cochlea and the hearing nerve.

Middle ear: the second section of the ear. We cannot see it. It contains three tiny bones.

Outer ear: the first section of the ear. It includes the pinna and the ear canal.

Pinna: the part of the outer ear that we can see. It catches sound.

Sound wave: how sound travels. Sound moves in waves that we cannot see.

Inside Your Ears

Everyone knows that our ears are for hearing. Our world is filled with thousands of sounds to hear. These sounds help us to learn about our world. We listen to sounds all day long, but we never think about what makes us hear them. When someone talks or a dog barks, do you ever wonder how you hear it?

Do you know what your ears look like? There is more to your ears than the part you can see. The most important part is inside the head. Here is what the whole ear would look like if you could see it:

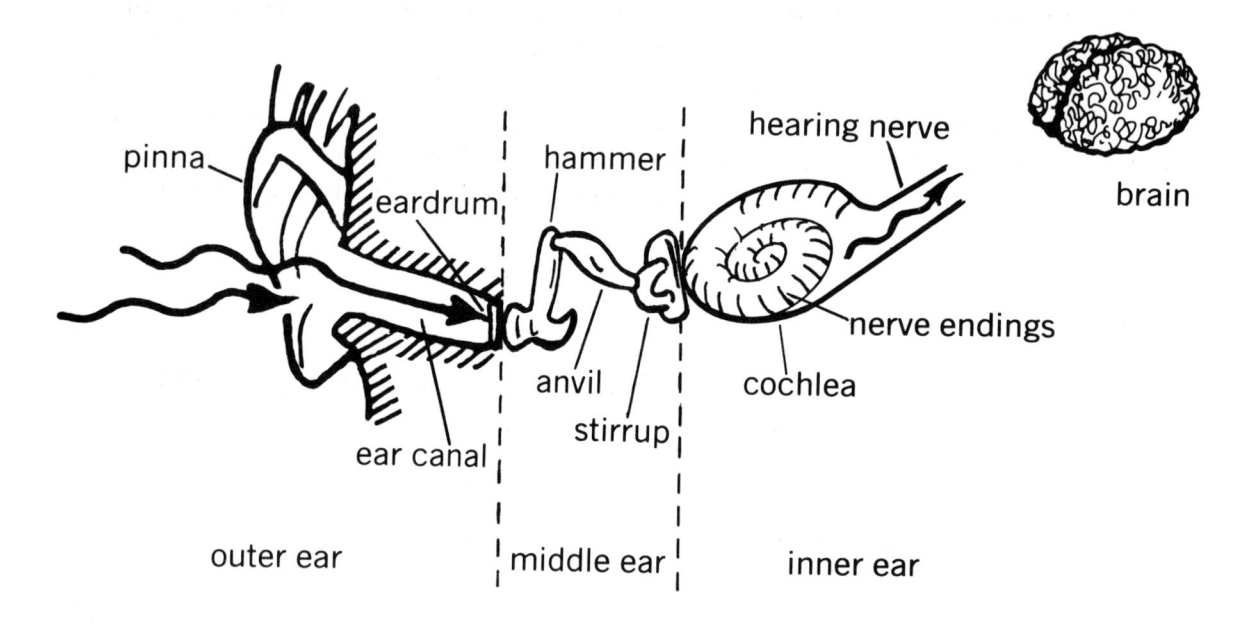

The Parts of the Ear

The **ear** is divided into three main sections: the outer ear, the middle ear, and the inner ear. Sound passes through all three sections of the ear before it goes to the brain. The brain interprets the sounds and tells us what we are hearing.

Sound goes into the **outer ear**. The part of the outer ear that we can see is called the **pinna**. It catches sound. Sound travels from the pinna through the **ear canal**. The sound pushes against our **eardrum**. The eardrum lies between the outer ear and the middle ear. It is a little opening covered with skin, kind of like a drum. Sound hits the eardrum and makes it vibrate (move back and forth).

The **middle ear** contains the three smallest bones in the body. These bones are called the **hammer**, the **anvil**, and the **stirrup** because of their shape. These bones are so small, they could fit on a dime. When the eardrum moves, it makes the three bones move.

The **inner ear** is deep inside your head. The inner ear contains the **cochlea** and the **hearing nerve**. The cochlea is shaped like a snail. It has thousands of tiny nerve endings inside it. These nerve endings lead to the hearing nerve. The nerve endings in the cochlea are tuned somewhat like the keys on a piano. Some of the nerve endings respond to low sounds, and some respond to high sounds. The hearing nerve connects the cochlea with the brain.

The three sections of the ear work together to help us hear. This is what happens: sounds hit the eardrum, so the eardrum starts to vibrate. The vibrations make the hammer, the anvil, and the stirrup move. This causes the nerve endings in the cochlea to move. The nerve endings send a message to the hearing nerve. The hearing nerve carries the message to the brain. The brain tells us what we are hearing. It tells us if we are hearing music, noise, a voice, a car horn, or a dog. That is how we hear!

EXERCISE 1

You have read much about your ears. Can you answer these questions? Check your answers with the Answer Key when you are finished.

1. Write T if the sentence is true. Write F if the sentence is false.

    a. _____ There are two bones inside our middle ear.

    b. _____ We can see the middle ear.

    c. _____ The pinna catches sound.

    d. _____ The cochlea is inside the middle ear.

    e. _____ Sounds hit against the eardrum and make it move.

    f. _____ The hammer, anvil, and stirrup are in the inner ear.

    g. _____ The hammer, anvil, and stirrup move.

    h. _____ The hearing nerve is inside the inner ear.

    i. _____ The nerve endings inside the cochlea do not move.

2. Fill in the blank with the correct answer.

   eardrum   hammer, anvil, and stirrup
   brain   ear canal
   cochlea   hearing nerve

   a. The _____ is filled with thousands of tiny nerve endings.

   b. The _____ is a tiny opening covered with skin.

   c. The _____ tells us what we are hearing.

   d. The _____ carries messages to the brain.

   e. The _____ are the three smallest bones in the body.

3. Write the name of each part of the ear next to its number.

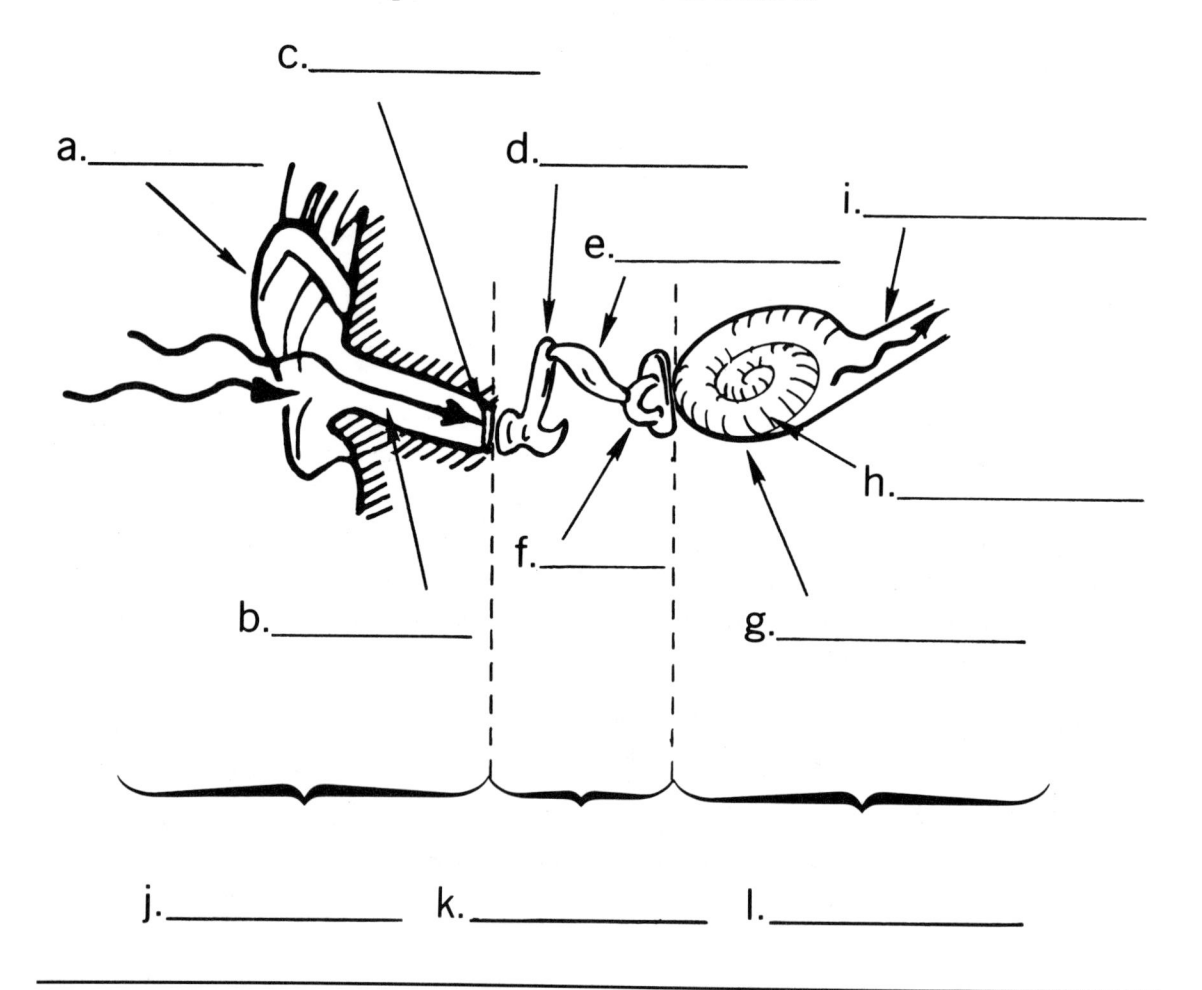

   a. _____
   b. _____
   c. _____
   d. _____
   e. _____
   f. _____
   g. _____
   h. _____
   i. _____
   j. _____
   k. _____
   l. _____

What Is Sound?

Our ears hear sound. Sound moves through the air. It moves in waves that we cannot see. This is what a **sound wave** would look like if we could see it:

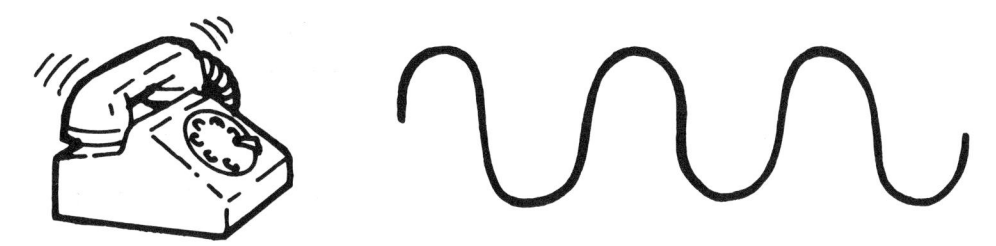

Sounds can be different from each other in many ways. A sound can be loud or soft. The loudness of a sound is measured in **decibels**. The decibel number tells us how loud or soft a sound is. If a sound has a low decibel number, then the sound is soft. If a sound has a high decibel number, the sound is loud.

Look at the chart. It shows how loud some sounds are. The loudness of the sounds is written in decibels. Look at the loudness of each sound. As the numbers get larger, the sounds get louder.

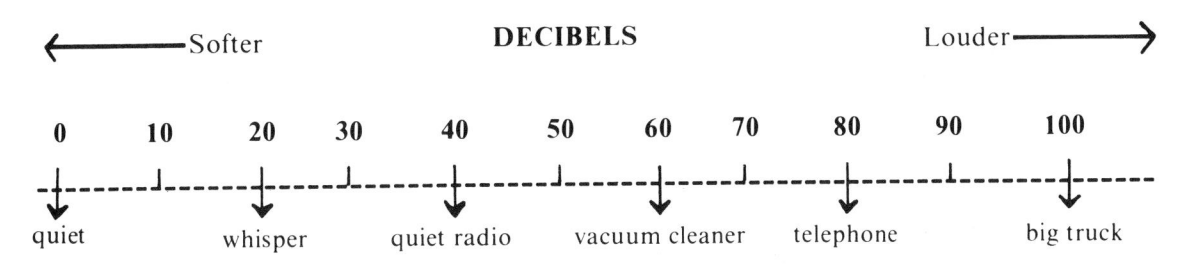

⟵——Softer   **DECIBELS**   Louder——⟶

| 0 | 10 | 20 | 30 | 40 | 50 | 60 | 70 | 80 | 90 | 100 |

quiet — whisper — quiet radio — vacuum cleaner — telephone — big truck

Sounds can be different in another way. A sound can be high or low. The **frequency** of a sound means how high or low the sound is. The frequency of a sound is measured in **hertz** (Hz).

Frequency is the number of sound waves that move through the air each second. A high sound has a high frequency. It has a high number of hertz. It sends many sound waves through the air each second. A whistle has a high frequency. The sound waves are close together and look like this:

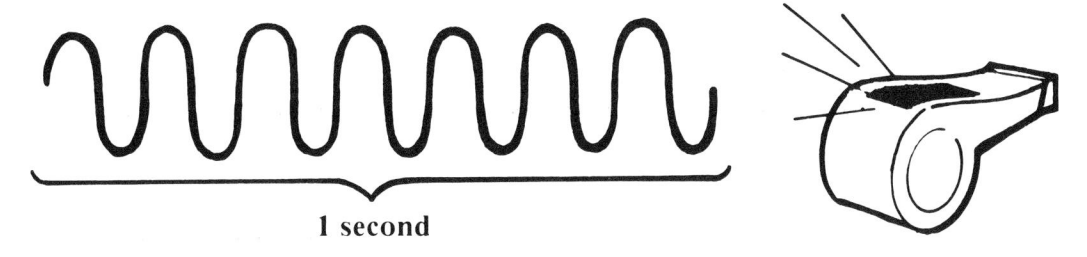

1 second

A low sound has a low frequency. It has a low number of hertz. It sends fewer sound waves through the air each second. A drum has a low frequency. The sound waves are far apart and look like this:

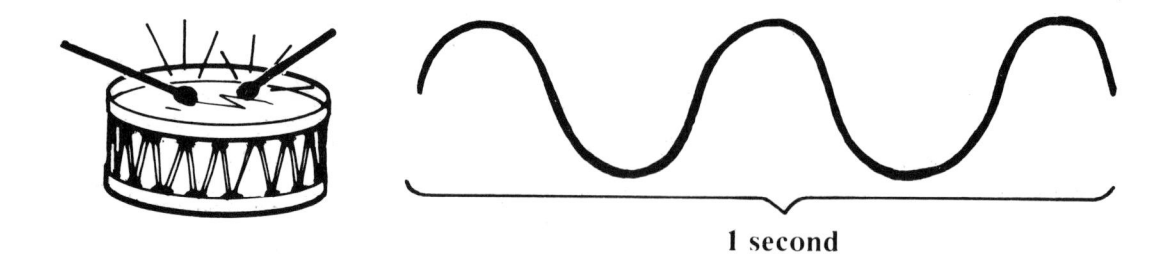

1 second

Our speech has different frequencies in it. All vowels have low frequency sounds. Examples are the *ee* in beet, the *u* in cup, and the *oo* in book. Some consonants have only high frequency sounds. Examples are the *th* in thumb, the *f* in fan, and the *s* in sun.

The next chart shows how high or low some sounds are. The frequency of the sounds is written as hertz. Look at the frequency of each sound. As the numbers get larger, the sounds get higher.

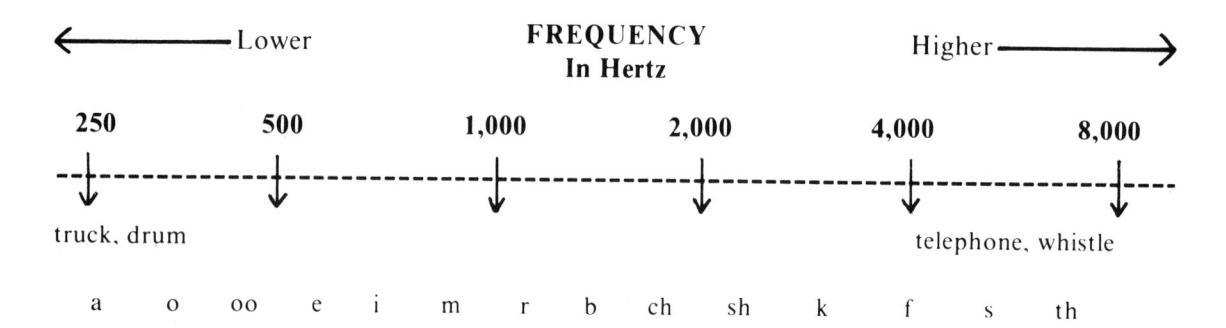

⟵──────Lower   **FREQUENCY**   Higher──────⟶
                      In Hertz

| 250 | 500 | 1,000 | 2,000 | 4,000 | 8,000 |

truck, drum   telephone, whistle

a   o   oo   e   i   m   r   b   ch   sh   k   f   s   th

EXERCISE 2

You have read much about sound. Can you answer these questions? Check your answers with the Answer Key when you are finished.

1. Circle each correct answer.

   a. What moves through the air?

      decibel   sound wave   frequency

10

b. What tells us how loud or soft a sound is?

        decibel   sound wave   frequency

c. What tells us how high or low a sound is?

        decibel   sound wave   frequency

d. Which sound is higher in decibels?

        a jet engine   a vacuum cleaner

e. Which sound has the higher frequency?

        the *e* in get   the *sh* in shoe

f. Can we see sound waves?

        yes   no

2. Fill in the blank with the correct answer.

   a. Sound moves through the air in _____.

        straight lines   waves   circles

   b. The frequency of a sound is how many sound waves move through the air each _____.

        second   minute   hour

   c. Sounds with a low frequency have sound waves that are _____.

        close together   double   far apart

   d. Most vowel sounds are _____ in frequency than consonant sounds.

        shorter   lower   higher

   e. The frequency of a sound is measured in _____.

        decibels   fractions   hertz

Lesson 2

Different Kinds of Hearing Loss

New Vocabulary

You will learn these words as you read this lesson. Say each word. Read its definition.

Buddy: a classmate who helps hearing-impaired students when they do not hear something. A buddy may also take notes during class for them.

Conductive hearing loss: a hearing loss caused by a problem in the outer ear or the middle ear.

Fluid: a watery liquid that can fill the middle ear. The fluid prevents the bones from moving.

Hearing aid: a small object that makes sounds and speech louder.

Hearing-impaired student: a student who has a hearing loss.

Mild hearing loss: soft sounds cannot be heard.

Mixed hearing loss: a hearing loss caused by a nerve loss and a conductive loss. There is a problem with the inner ear. There is also a problem with the outer ear or middle ear.

Moderate hearing loss: sounds cannot be heard until they become fairly loud.

Nerve loss: a hearing loss caused by a problem with the nerve endings in the inner ear.

Profound hearing loss: no sounds can be heard.

Severe hearing loss: only very loud sounds can be heard.

Special classroom seating: the best seats in a classroom for hearing-impaired students. It helps them hear and see what the teacher and other students are saying.

Speechreading: a way to understand what someone is saying by watching the person's face, mouth, and body movements.

Types of Hearing Loss

Something may go wrong with our ears that causes us to lose some of our hearing. Many people have a hearing loss. There are three types of hearing loss: conductive, nerve, and mixed.

Conductive Hearing Loss

A **conductive hearing loss** means something is wrong with the outer ear or the middle ear. The outer ear or the middle ear can become damaged (hurt) in many ways. Here are some of the ways.

1. A baby can be born with a conductive loss.
    a. A baby can be born without a pinna, an eardrum, or bones inside the ear.
    b. A baby can be born with a damaged ear canal. If the ear canal is blocked, sound waves cannot travel to the eardrum.
2. Sharp objects, like pencils or hairpins, can put a hole in the eardrum. (Never put sharp objects in your ears!)
3. Loud noises, like from a firecracker or an explosion, can create a hole in the eardrum.
4. Getting hit on the head very hard can damage the middle ear.
5. The three bones in the middle ear, which are hooked together by tiny muscles, can grow together. When this happens, the bones cannot move easily. That prevents sound waves from reaching the inner ear.
6. Germs from a cold or sickness can get into the middle ear.
    a. The germs can damage the tiny bones.
    b. The germs may make the middle ear fill up with **fluid** (a watery liquid). The bones cannot move easily when there is fluid inside the middle ear. Many children have fluid in their ears. That is why they have tubes in their ears. The tubes drain the fluid from their ears.

Doctors can help many people with a conductive loss to hear better. Doctors can give a person a new pinna, ear canal, or eardrum. They can patch a hole in the eardrum. If the bones have grown together, a doctor can take them apart so they move easily again.

Nerve Loss

A **nerve loss** is caused by a problem in the inner ear. It is called a nerve loss because the nerve endings in the inner ear are damaged. Doctors do not always know what causes a nerve loss. But sometimes the doctors do know. Here are some of the causes of nerve loss.

1. A baby can be born with a nerve loss.
    a. Someone in the baby's family may have a hearing loss; it can be passed to the new baby.

b. The baby's mother might have been sick or might have taken some harmful medicine while she was pregnant. The sickness or medicine could have damaged the nerve endings in the baby's cochlea.

2. A baby can be born too early. Babies who are born too early often get sick because they are so little. They may have a high fever or have trouble breathing. These things can damage the nerve endings in a baby's inner ear.

3. A person can get nerve damage from a high fever. A high fever can damage the nerve endings in the ear. Mumps, measles, chicken pox, and the flu can cause a high fever. These sicknesses can cause a nerve loss. Sometimes the medicine a person takes while sick can damage the nerve endings.

4. Getting hit on the head very hard can hurt the inner ear.

5. Loud noises, like loud music, can destroy the nerve endings in the inner ear.

6. Many older people have trouble hearing. The nerve endings in their ears lose some of the ability to send sound messages to the brain.

Doctors cannot help people with a nerve loss. Doctors cannot fix damaged nerves. That is why a person with a nerve loss will always have a hearing problem.

Mixed Hearing Loss

Some people have both a nerve loss and a conductive loss. This is called a **mixed hearing loss**. A mixed loss means there is damage to the inner ear and to the middle or outer ear.

EXERCISE 3

You have read much about the types of hearing loss. Can you answer these questions? Check your answers with the Answer Key when you are finished.

1. Give two causes of a conductive hearing loss.

2. Give two causes of a nerve loss.

3. Match the words that go together by drawing lines between them.

   Kind of loss   *Damaged part*

   a. mixed loss   inner ear

   b. conductive loss   outer, middle, and inner ear

   c. nerve loss   outer ear and middle ear

4. Write T if the sentence is true. Write F if the sentence is false.

   a. _____ Fluid can fill the middle ear.

   b. _____ There is no way to drain fluid from the ear.

   c. _____ Doctors can fix damaged nerve endings.

   d. _____ Doctors can help people with a conductive loss.

   e. _____ Doctors can help people with a nerve loss.

Levels of Hearing Loss

Everyone does not have the same amount of hearing loss. Some people have less hearing than other people. There are four different levels of hearing loss: mild, moderate, severe, and profound.

People with a **mild hearing loss** cannot hear soft sounds. Sometimes they have to ask other people to repeat what they've said. It is hard for them to hear in noisy places.

A **moderate hearing loss** means that sounds must be fairly loud before a person can hear them. People with a moderate loss have trouble hearing others talk unless they talk loudly. Speech may not sound clear to them.

People with a **severe hearing loss** can hear only very loud sounds. They cannot hear others talk. Many speech sounds are not clear to them. People with a severe loss hear vowels better than consonants.

Even very loud sounds are not heard by people with a **profound hearing loss**. They cannot hear speech even if someone shouts. Low sounds, such as vowels, may be the only sounds they can hear. People with a profound loss may hear sounds only by feeling them through the body.

A person can have the same hearing loss in each ear. For example, a person may have a moderate loss in the right ear and the left ear. But many people have a different loss in each ear. For example, a person can have a mild loss in the right ear and a severe loss in the left ear.

Many people have a hearing problem for their whole life. Doctors or medicine cannot help them hear better. A **hearing aid** is the only thing that helps them. The hearing aid makes sounds louder. It makes sounds loud enough for these people to hear. The aid helps them to hear sounds that they could not hear before.

Most people with a hearing loss have some hearing that they can use. They can hear some sounds even without a hearing aid. They may be able to hear some sounds, but they cannot hear all sounds. The sounds they hear may be different from what others hear.

EXERCISE 4

You have read much about the levels of hearing loss. Can you answer these questions? Check your answers with the Answer Key when you are finished.

1. Fill in the blank with the correct answer.

    A. mild loss   C. severe loss
    B. moderate loss   D. profound loss

    a. _____ The person can hear sounds that are fairly loud.

    b. _____ The person cannot hear speech, even if the speaker shouts.

    c. _____ Sounds must be very loud before the person hears them.

    d. _____ Soft sounds may be the only sounds the person cannot hear.

2. Write T if the sentence is true. Write F if the sentence is false.

    a. _____ Everyone has the same level of hearing loss.

    b. _____ A person always has the same loss in both ears.

    c. _____ Most people can hear some sounds, even without a hearing aid.

    d. _____ Someone with a profound loss has better hearing than someone with a moderate loss.

3. What does a hearing aid do? Put a check in front of each correct answer. Find two answers.

    A hearing aid:

    a. _____ helps people see better.

b. _____ helps people hear better.

c. _____ helps people swim faster.

d. _____ makes people hungry.

e. _____ makes sounds shorter.

f. _____ makes sounds louder.

Hearing-Impaired Students

A **hearing-impaired student** is a student who has a hearing loss. Some students who cannot hear well may have trouble learning in school. Reading, spelling, or English grammar may be very hard for them. They may have trouble hearing films in school. Hearing-impaired students may not always hear what their teachers or other students say. Understanding directions may be hard for them. They may not know the meanings of many words. They may have trouble putting words together to make sentences.

A hearing loss can cause some students to have speech problems. Hearing-impaired students may have speech problems if they cannot hear some sounds clearly. Sounds that may be hard for them to say are: *s, z, sh, ch, f,* and *th*. These sounds are hard to hear because they have a high frequency.

A hearing aid helps most students with a hearing loss. A hearing aid makes sounds and speech louder. An aid helps hearing-impaired students to hear their teachers and classmates better. Hearing-impaired students must learn how to wear a hearing aid and how to take care of it. They must learn to listen to sounds through the hearing aid. They must learn to tell the difference between a dog barking, a bell ringing, or a person talking. They must learn to tell the difference between words that sound alike, such as *mat* and *bat*.

Students with a hearing loss often read lips to understand speech. **Speechreading** helps these students know what someone is saying. Hearing-impaired students learn to watch a speaker's face, body movements, and mouth movements. They learn the lip and tongue movements that go with each sound. They learn that facial expressions and movements can help them understand what a speaker is talking about.

Special classroom seating is helpful to students with a hearing loss. Special classroom seating is the best seat in the classroom for hearing-impaired students. It helps them to hear and see what their teachers or classmates are saying. Special seating is always close to the speaker. It helps hearing-impaired students hear the speaker's voice more easily. It also helps them see the speaker's face clearly for speechreading.

The best place for hearing-impaired students to sit is toward the front of the room. The better ear should face the teacher and other students. This will make listening easier. Sitting toward one side of the room makes it easier to speechread everyone in the room.

Many students with a hearing loss have a **buddy** in their classroom. A buddy is a classmate who helps out in many ways. The buddy helps hearing-impaired students when they do not hear announcements. The buddy may repeat what the teacher or other students say during class. Then the students with a hearing loss do not miss important things. The students do not miss assignments or directions. They know when there will be a test. They know which page to turn to during class. They know important names, dates, or vocabulary words. A buddy can be very helpful with all of these things.

Sometimes students must take notes during class. This is very hard for the students with a hearing loss. They cannot take notes, speechread, and listen to the teacher all at the same time! This is where a buddy can be especially helpful. A buddy can take notes for the hearing-impaired students. Then the students can speechread the teacher and listen better. They have more time to think about what the teacher is saying. The buddy gives a copy of the notes to the students after class.

Students with a hearing loss should always tell their teachers about it. The teachers may not know about the hearing loss, or they may forget about it.

A teacher can be very helpful to students with a hearing loss. The teacher can do things that make it easier for these students to hear. Here are some of the things the teacher can do.

1. The teacher can speak loudly and clearly.
2. The teacher can repeat directions or assignments if the students did not hear them.
3. The teacher can write important things on the chalkboard so the students *see* them.
4. The teacher can stand still while talking so the students can speechread better.
5. The teacher can stand close to the students while talking so they can hear better.
6. The teacher can give the students special classroom seating to help them hear and see others.
7. The teacher can let a buddy help the students.
8. The teacher can talk about a film before showing it so the students understand it better.

EXERCISE 5

You have read much about hearing-impaired students. Can you answer these questions? Check your answers with the Answer Key when you are finished.

1. Which of these sentences are true about speechreading? Put a check in front of each correct answer. Find three answers.

   a. _____ Speechreading means watching a person's mouth.

   b. _____ Speechreading means watching a person's feet.

   c. _____ Speechreading means watching a person's body movements.

   d. _____ Speechreading helps a person to know what others are saying.

   e. _____ Speechreading is easy when the speaker mumbles words.

   f. _____ Speechreading is easy when the speaker's back is turned.

2. What is special classroom seating? Put a check in front of each correct answer. Find six answers.

   Special classroom seating is:

   a. _____ a seat far away from the speaker.

   b. _____ a seat close to the speaker.

   c. _____ a seat where the student can hear and see others easily.

   d. _____ a seat that makes speechreading easier.

   e. _____ a seat that makes sleeping easier.

   f. _____ a seat that makes listening easier.

   g. _____ a seat toward the back of the room.

   h. _____ a seat toward the front of the room.

   i. _____ a seat close to the teacher.

3. What can hearing-impaired students do to hear better in school? Put a check in front of each correct answer. Find six answers.

   Hearing-impaired students can:

   a. _____ wear a hearing aid.

   b. _____ wear brown shoes.

c. ____ have special classroom seating.

d. ____ speechread.

e. ____ look at the floor when people talk.

f. ____ sit in the back of the room.

g. ____ tell every teacher about their hearing loss.

h. ____ ask a buddy for help when they don't hear something.

i. ____ sleep during class.

j. ____ sit with their better ear facing the teacher and other students.

4. Which things can make it hard for a hearing-impaired student to speechread or listen in the classroom? Put a check in front of each correct answer. Find nine answers.

   It is hard to speechread or listen when:

   a. ____ there is noise from chairs scraping, people coughing, the heater clanging, etc.

   b. ____ the teacher talks while writing on the chalkboard.

   c. ____ the speaker covers his or her mouth with a hand or a book.

   d. ____ the speaker talks loudly and clearly.

   e. ____ several students are talking at the same time.

   f. ____ the teacher talks while moving around the room.

   g. ____ the teacher writes important things on the chalkboard.

   h. ____ a teacher or student mumbles while talking.

   i. ____ a film does not show the speaker who is talking.

   j. ____ the classroom is quiet.

   k. ____ the student must take notes while the teacher is talking.

   l. ____ the student sits far away from the speaker.

Lesson 3

How Hearing Is Tested

New Vocabulary

You will learn these words as you read this lesson. Say each word. Read its definition.

Audiogram: a chart that shows how well a person hears sounds.

Audiologist: a person who tests hearing and works with hearing-impaired people.

Audiology clinic: a place where people can have their hearing tested. An audiology clinic sells and fixes hearing aids, too.

Audiometer: a machine that tests hearing.

Earphones: a set of earphones are placed over the ears during a hearing test. They carry sounds from the audiometer to the ears.

Speech discrimination test: a test that shows how well a person hears the different vowel and consonant sounds in a word. The audiologist talks loud enough for the person to hear easily during this test.

Speech reception threshold test: a test that shows how loud speech must be before a person understands half of the words. The audiologist begins the test in a loud voice. Then the audiologist speaks softer and softer until the person cannot repeat the words anymore.

Threshold: the softest sounds that a person can hear during a hearing test.

Why Should You Have a Hearing Test?

A person's hearing can change from year to year. Some people's hearing can get worse without them even knowing it. That is why it is important for everyone to have a hearing test once in a while.

People can go to an **audiologist** for a hearing test. An audiologist is a person who works with hearing-impaired people. Many audiologists work in an **audiology clinic**. An audiology clinic is a place where people can have their hearing tested. An audiology clinic sells and fixes hearing aids, too.

Hearing-impaired people should have a hearing test every year. There are many reasons for this.

1. A hearing test will show if the person's hearing has changed or stayed the same.
2. The audiologist will check the earmold to see if it fits well. The earmold may be too small if the person's ear has grown. If the earmold is too old or cracked, the person will need to get a new earmold.
3. The audiologist will put the hearing aid into a special machine. The machine will test the aid to see if it is working well. The machine will show if the aid needs to be fixed.
4. The audiologist may want to try a different hearing aid on the person's ear. A different aid may help the person to hear even better than the aid the person has.

The Audiogram

Your hearing can be tested with a machine called an **audiometer**. The audiometer makes sounds at different frequencies. The sounds can be high or low. The audiometer also makes the sounds at different decibels. The sounds can be loud or soft.

A set of **earphones** goes on your head. The earphones cover your ears. They carry sounds from the audiometer to your ears. Each time you hear a sound, you raise your hand.

During the hearing test, the audiologist usually tests these frequencies: 250, 500, 1000, 2000, 4000, and 8000. The higher the number, the higher the frequency of the sound. The audiologist tests each frequency at different loudness levels. At first the sounds are very loud. The audiometer can make sounds up to 110 decibels. Then the sounds become softer and softer until you cannot hear them. The softest sound that you can hear is called your **threshold**.

The frequencies of 500, 1000, and 2000 Hz are very important. Those are the frequencies of almost all the speech sounds. A person who has trouble hearing the frequencies of 500, 1000, and 2000 Hz will have trouble hearing speech sounds.

The audiologist writes on a chart how well you hear the test sounds. This chart is called an **audiogram**. The audiogram shows how well you hear sounds. Look at Figure 1. It is an audiogram. Look at the different frequencies. Look at the different decibels.

The audiologist writes Os and Xs on the audiogram. The Os show how well the right ear hears. The Xs show how well the left ear hears. The audiogram shows how loud a sound must be before each ear can hear it.

Many people can hear a sound at 0 decibels. They have very good hearing. They do not have a hearing loss. All of their Os and Xs are near the top of the audiogram.

Not everyone has good hearing. The Os and Xs are not always near the top of the audiogram. Some people cannot hear a frequency until it is much louder than 0 decibels. If a person can only hear a frequency at 50 decibels or louder, that person's threshold is 50 decibels.

You already know about the different levels of hearing loss. A person can have a mild, a moderate, a severe, or a profound hearing loss. The audiologist figures out a person's hearing loss by looking at the person's threshold at different frequencies. That's why the audiologist can describe a hearing loss in decibels (for example, a 40 decibel loss). Look at the chart.

Loudness of Sounds	Level of Hearing Loss
20–40 decibels	mild loss
40–60 decibels	moderate loss
60–90 decibels	severe loss
90–110 decibels	profound loss

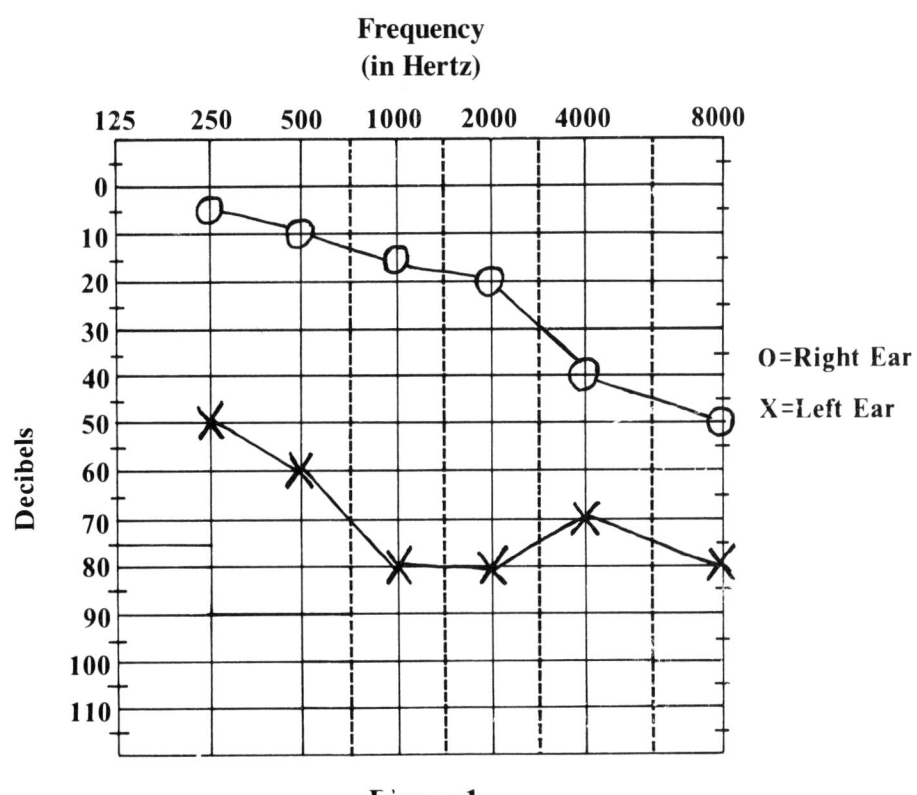

Figure 1
A Sample Audiogram

EXERCISE 6

You have read much about an audiogram. Can you answer these questions? Check your answers with the Answer Key when you are finished.

1. Match the words that go together by drawing lines between them.

    a. a person who tests hearing   an audiogram

    b. a chart of how well a person can hear   an audiometer

    c. a machine that tests hearing   an audiology clinic

    d. a place that does hearing tests   an audiologist

2. Write T if the sentence is true. Write F if the sentence is false.

    a. _____ An audiologist tests hearing.

    b. _____ A person's hearing cannot change.

    c. _____ The frequencies of 6000, 7000, and 8000 are very important for hearing speech sounds.

    d. _____ Earphones carry sounds from the audiometer to the ears.

    e. _____ People with normal hearing never need to have a hearing test.

3. How often should your hearing be tested?

    a. _____ once a week

    b. _____ once a month

    c. _____ once a year

4. Why is it important to have your hearing tested each year? Put a check in front of each correct answer. Find four answers.

    I should have my hearing tested each year to see if:

    a. _____ my hearing has changed.

    b. _____ I need a new earmold.

    c. _____ my hearing aid is working well.

    d. _____ I have grown taller.

    e. _____ I need new batteries.

f. ____ a different hearing aid might be better for me than the one I now have.

g. ____ I need glasses.

5. Match the words that go together by drawing lines between them.

    a. 20–40 decibels   moderate hearing loss

    b. 40–60 decibels   profound hearing loss

    c. 60–90 decibels   mild hearing loss

    d. 90–110 decibels   severe hearing loss

6. Which of these would you find on an audiogram? Put a check in front of each correct answer. Find four answers.

    a. ____ some Xs   d. ____ different frequencies

    b. ____ some Rs   e. ____ different decibels

    c. ____ some Os   f. ____ different flowers

7. Which of these sentences are true about an audiogram? Put a check in front of each correct answer. Find three answers.

    a. ____ It shows how well a person dances.

    b. ____ It shows how well a person hears sounds.

    c. ____ It is done with an audiometer.

    d. ____ It is done by a dentist.

    e. ____ It shows how loud a frequency must be before the ear can hear it.

8. Turn back to the audiogram on page 23. Look at it as you answer these questions. Answer the questions by writing either "right ear" or "left ear" in the blanks.

    a. Which ear can hear better? _____

    b. Which ear has a severe hearing loss? _____

    c. Which ear has trouble hearing speech sounds? _____

    d. Which ear should be facing a speaker so the person can hear better? _____

    e. Which ear cannot hear low frequencies easily? _____

Tests for Hearing Speech

The audiologist needs to know how well a person hears and understands words. The audiologist can test hearing for speech with an audiometer. The audiologist may speak into a microphone or play a record that has words on it. Earphones carry the words from the audiometer to the ears.

The audiologist will test how loud words must be before you can understand what is said. The audiologist wants to know how loud people must talk before you understand them. This test is called a **speech reception threshold test**. The audiologist says words (like *airplane, sidewalk,* or *birthday*) to find your speech reception threshold score.

The audiologist begins the test with a loud voice, then says the words softer and softer. The speech reception threshold is the loudness at which you can understand half of the words on the test. That is why it is marked in decibels. The speech reception threshold score can be between 0 and 100 decibels. A score close to 0 decibels means a person has no trouble understanding speech.

The audiologist will also test how well you can hear the different sounds in a word. This is called the **speech discrimination test**. Every word has vowel and consonant sounds in it. Some consonants sound alike; for example, *p* and *b, t* and *d,* and *c* and *g*. That's why some words sound alike; for example, *pet* and *bet, toe* and *dough,* and *could* and *good*.

The audiologist finds your speech discrimination score by saying short words like *rat, sled,* and *box*. You must repeat the words. Your score is the percentage of words you repeat correctly. The score can be between 0 and 100. A score close to 100% means a person can easily hear different vowel and consonant sounds.

EXERCISE 7

You have read much about tests for hearing speech. Can you answer these questions? Check your answers with the Answer Key when you are finished.

1. Which of these sentences are true about the speech reception threshold test? Put a check in front of each correct answer. Find seven answers.

    a. _____ It is done with an audiometer.

    b. _____ It is done by an audiologist.

    c. _____ It shows how well a person understands music.

    d. _____ It shows how well a person understands speech.

    e. _____ Words like *baseball* are used.

f. _____ It shows how much a person weighs.

g. _____ The score is marked in pounds.

h. _____ The score is marked in decibels.

i. _____ It shows how loud words must be before the person understands them.

j. _____ It shows how old a person is.

k. _____ A score close to 0 decibels means the person understands speech well.

l. _____ A score close to 85 decibels means the person understands speech well.

2. Which of these sentences are true about the speech discrimination test? Put a check in front of each correct answer. Find seven answers.

    a. _____ Words like *please* are used.

    b. _____ It shows how well a person can do math homework.

    c. _____ It shows how tall a person is.

    d. _____ The score is marked in inches.

    e. _____ The score is marked as the percentage correct.

    f. _____ It shows how well a person hears a piano.

    g. _____ It shows how well a person hears speech.

    h. _____ A score close to 20% means the person can hear speech easily.

    i. _____ A score close to 100% means the person can hear speech easily.

    j. _____ It shows how well the person hears different vowel and consonant sounds.

    k. _____ It is done with an audiometer.

    l. _____ It is done by an audiologist.

Lesson 4

Understanding Your Audiogram

How You Hear Sounds

You have learned how hearing is tested for sounds and for speech. Now you are ready to write down the results of your tests. This will help you to understand how well you hear sounds and speech. It will help you to understand why you must wear a hearing aid.

You will need a copy of your audiogram to do this section. Ask your audiologist for a copy of your audiogram. It should only be one or two years old.

Look at the blank audiogram on page 29. This will be your audiogram. Fill in the audiogram to show how well you hear sounds. Follow these directions for your audiogram.

1. Look at the audiogram from your audiologist. Look at the Os marked on it. The Os show how well your right ear hears. Copy each O onto the blank audiogram. Be sure to mark each O in the correct place. Connect the Os with a line.
2. Look at the audiogram again. Look at the Xs marked on it. The Xs show how well your left ear hears. Copy each X onto the blank audiogram. Be sure to mark each X in the correct place. Connect the Xs with a line.

You have copied many Os and Xs. Do you know what they mean? They show how well each ear can hear. For example, an O or an X at 45 decibels means that your ear cannot hear that sound until it is 45 decibels loud.

Very good hearing is at 0 decibels on the audiogram. That is at the top of the audiogram. Are any of your Os or Xs close to 0 decibels? This means your ear can hear some sounds easily. Your ear can hear well if most Os and Xs are close to 0 decibels. Your ear can hear soft sounds.

Are any of your Os or Xs toward the bottom of the audiogram? This means your ear has trouble hearing some sounds. Your ear has much trouble hearing if most Os or Xs are toward the bottom of the audiogram. Sounds must be very loud before you can hear them.

Both of your ears may hear the same. If so, the Os and Xs are close to each other on your audiogram. Or, one ear may hear better than the other ear. The Os and Xs are not close to each other.

**Frequency
(in Hertz)**

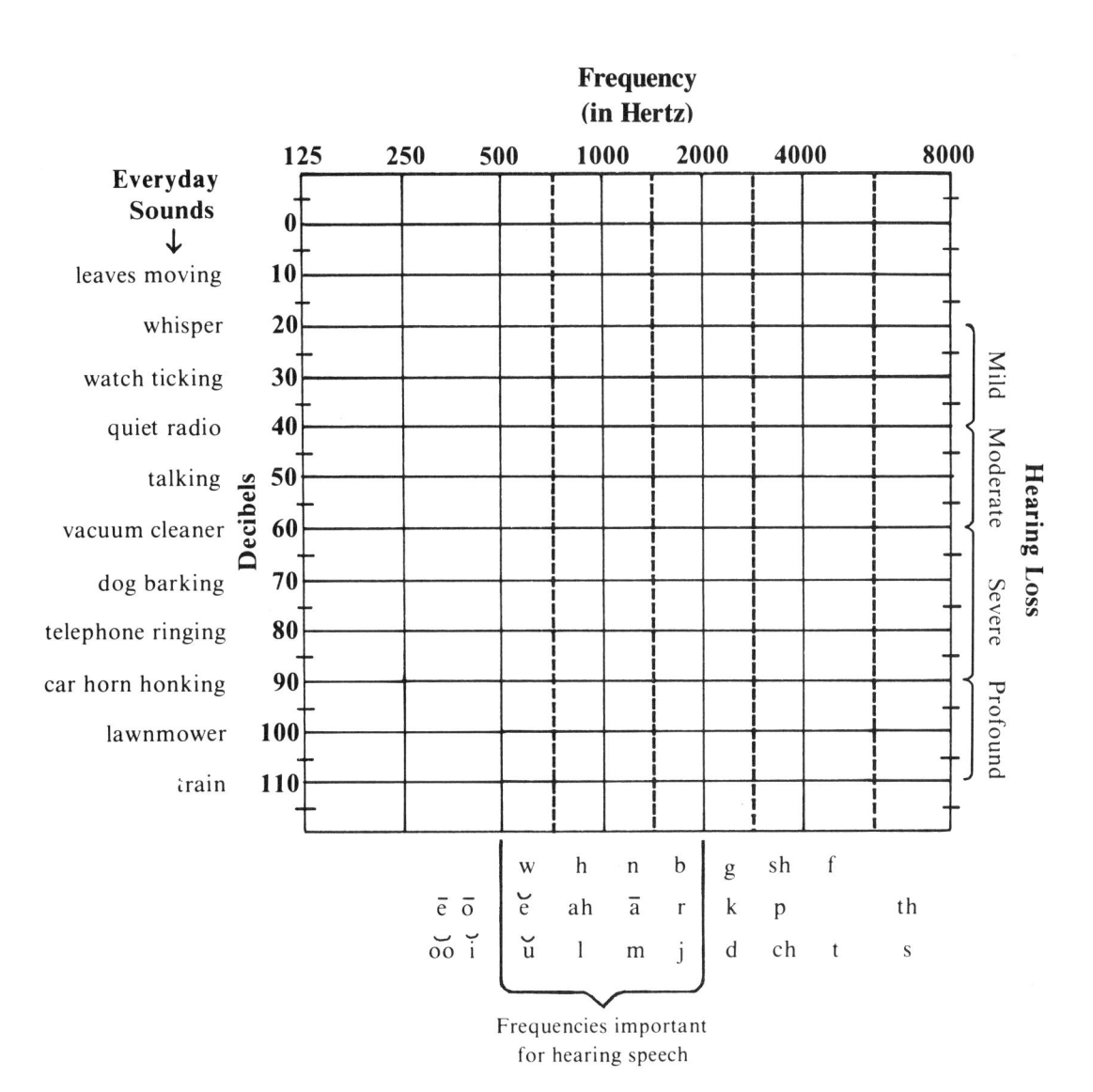

	125	250	500	1000	2000	4000	8000

Everyday Sounds ↓

Sound	Decibels
leaves moving	10
whisper	20
watch ticking	30
quiet radio	40
talking	50
vacuum cleaner	60
dog barking	70
telephone ringing	80
car horn honking	90
lawnmower	100
train	110

Hearing Loss: Mild, Moderate, Severe, Profound

	w	h	n	b	g	sh	f
ē ō	ĕ	ah	ā	r	k	p	th
ŏŏ ĭ	ŭ	l	m	j	d	ch	t	s

Frequencies important for hearing speech

O = Right Ear   X = Left Ear

29

**Frequency
(in Hertz)**

EXERCISE 8

Look carefully at your audiogram. Think about what the Os and Xs mean. Then answer these questions about your hearing. Everyone will have different answers to these questions. The answers are not in the Answer Key. Show your answers to your teacher.

1. Which ear has a hearing loss? Put a check in front of the correct answer.

    a. ____ Only my right ear has a hearing loss (many Os are louder than 20 decibels; all the Xs are close to 0 decibels).

    b. ____ Only my left ear has a hearing loss (many Xs are louder than 20 decibels; all the Os are close to 0 decibels).

    c. ____ Both ears have a hearing loss (many Os and Xs are louder than 20 decibels).

2. Which ear can hear better? Put a check in front of the correct answer.

    a. ____ My right ear can hear better (many Os are above the Xs).

    b. ____ My left ear can hear better (many Xs are above the Os).

    c. ____ Both ears hear about the same (all the Os and Xs are close to each other).

3. Look on the left side of your audiogram. Many sounds you hear every day are given. Each sound is next to a decibel number. The decibel number tells how loud the sound is. High decibel numbers mean the sounds are loud.

    a. Name the sounds that are loud enough for you to hear easily without a hearing aid.

    b. Name the sounds that you have trouble hearing without a hearing aid.

4. Many vowels and consonants are written at the bottom of your audiogram. Vowel sounds usually have low frequencies. They are written toward the left side of the audiogram. Consonant sounds usually have high frequencies. They are written toward the right side of the audiogram.

   a. Name the vowels and consonants you can hear easily without a hearing aid.

   b. Name the vowels and consonants you have trouble hearing without a hearing aid.

5. Look at the frequencies of 250, 500, and 1000 Hz. They are lower frequencies. A drum has a low frequency. Look at the frequencies of 2000, 4000, and 8000 Hz. They are high frequencies. A whistle has a high frequency.

   a. Which does your right ear hear better (where are the Os closer to 0 decibels)?

   ____ the lower frequencies

   ____ the higher frequencies

   ____ my right ear hears low and high frequencies about the same

   b. Which does your left ear hear better (where are the Xs closer to 0 decibels)?

   ____ the lower frequencies

   ____ the higher frequencies

   ____ my left ear hears low and high frequencies about the same

Your Hearing Loss

The frequencies of 500, 1000, and 2000 Hz are very important. These frequencies contain the speech sounds. How you hear these frequencies tells you about your hearing loss.

Look on the right side of the audiogram. You will see "Hearing Loss" written. The audiogram is divided into four areas: mild loss, moderate loss, severe loss, and profound loss.

Read the chart below. You have seen it before. It shows how loud the frequencies of 500, 1000, and 2000 Hz must be at each level of hearing loss.

Loudness of 500, 1000, & 2000 Hz	Level of Hearing Loss
20–40 decibels	mild loss
40–60 decibels	moderate loss
60–90 decibels	severe loss
90–110 decibels	profound loss

What level of hearing loss do you have in the right ear? What level of hearing loss do you have in the left ear? Follow these directions to find out.

Turn back to your audiogram. Look at the Os (right ear) for the frequencies of 500, 1000, and 2000 Hz. Look at the Xs (left ear) for the frequencies of 500, 1000, and 2000 Hz. How loud are these frequencies before each ear hears them? Write the numbers in the blanks.

Right ear = _____, _____, _____ decibels

Left ear = _____, _____, _____ decibels

When these frequencies are inside the area of mild loss, you have a mild hearing loss in that ear. Your ear hears these frequencies at 20 to 40 decibels of loudness.

When these frequencies are inside the area of moderate loss, you have a moderate hearing loss in that ear. Your ear hears these frequencies at 40 to 60 decibels of loudness.

When these frequencies are inside the area of severe loss, you have a severe hearing loss in that ear. Your ear hears these frequencies at 60 to 90 decibels of loudness.

If these frequencies are inside the area of profound loss, then you have a profound hearing loss. The ear hears these frequencies when they are louder than 90 decibels.

An ear can have more than one amount of hearing loss. For example, an ear may have a mild loss at the frequency of 500 Hz. It may have a moderate loss at the frequencies of 1000 and 2000 Hz. When this happens, we say the ear has a mild-to-moderate loss. It has *both* amounts of hearing loss.

EXERCISE 9

What is your hearing loss? Find the frequencies of 500, 1000, and 2000 Hz on your audiogram. Then answer these questions. Everyone will have different answers to these questions. The answers are not in the Answer Key. Show your answers to your teacher.

1. What amount of hearing loss do you have in the right ear? Put a check in front of the correct answer. You may check more than one answer.

    a. _____ mild (the Os are inside the area of mild loss)

    b. _____ moderate (the Os are inside the area of moderate loss)

    c. _____ severe (the Os are inside the area of severe loss)

    d. _____ profound (the Os are inside the area of profound loss)

2. What amount of hearing loss do you have in the left ear? Put a check in front of the correct answer. You may check more than one answer.

    a. _____ mild (the Xs are inside the area of mild loss)

    b. _____ moderate (the Xs are inside the area of moderate loss)

    c. _____ severe (the Xs are inside the area of severe loss)

    d. _____ profound (the Xs are inside the area of profound loss)

3. Do both ears have the same amount of hearing loss? Put a check in front of the correct answer.

    a. _____ Yes (Both ears hear about the same.)

    b. _____ No (My ears do not hear the same.)

How You Hear Speech

Look at the audiogram from your audiologist. Below the audiogram is a section that shows how well you hear and understand speech. Find your speech reception threshold score on the audiogram. The score is written in decibels. It shows how loud words must be before you understand half of them. Copy your speech reception threshold score for each ear here:

Right ear = _____ decibels   Left ear = _____ decibels

What does this score mean? The *smaller* the number, the better your score. For example, a score of 32 decibels means you heard half of the words when they were 32 decibels loud. That is better than a score of 54 decibels. It means speech does not have to be as loud before you can understand it.

Look at your audiogram again. Find the section on speech discrimination. Your speech discrimination is how well you can hear different vowel and consonant sounds. Your speech discrimination score shows the percentage of words you repeated correctly. Copy your speech discrimination score for each ear here:

Right ear = _____%   Left ear = _____%

What does this score mean? The *larger* the number, the better your score. A score of 90% to 100% means that you have no trouble hearing different vowel or consonant sounds. A score of 76% to 88% means you have some trouble hearing the difference between sounds that are almost the same. You probably have trouble understanding what people tell you. For example, you may not be sure whether the audiologist said *me* or *knee, hot* or *hop, fin* or *thin*. A score of 75% or poorer means that you have much trouble understanding words. Speechreading may be the only thing that helps you to understand speech better. Even a hearing aid may not help you to understand speech. The hearing aid makes speech loud enough for you to hear, but it cannot help you to tell the difference between sounds that are almost the same.

EXERCISE 10

Look at the scores you have written. Think about what they mean. Then answer these questions about how well you hear and understand speech. Everyone will have different answers to these questions. The answers are not in the Answer Key. Show your answers to your teacher.

1. Which ear has the better (smaller) speech reception threshold score? Put a check in front of the correct answer.

    a. _____ my right ear (Its score is the smaller number.)

    b. _____ my left ear (Its score is the smaller number.)

    c. _____ both ears hear the same (They have the same score.)

2. Which ear has the better (larger) speech discrimination score? Put a check in front of the correct answer.

    a. _____ my right ear (Its score is the larger number.)

b. ____ my left ear (Its score is the larger number.)

c. ____ both ears hear the same (They have the same score.)

3. Is your speech discrimination score better or poorer than 75%?

    a. For the right ear:

    ____ better (A hearing aid can help me to hear speech better.)

    ____ poorer (A hearing aid may not help me to hear speech better.)

    b. For the left ear:

    ____ better (A hearing aid can help me to hear speech better.)

    ____ poorer (A hearing aid may not help me to hear speech better.)

Lesson 5

Questions About Your Hearing

There are many questions about your hearing in this section. The answers to these questions are important. They will help you to learn more about your hearing loss. They will help you to understand why you need a hearing aid.

These questions will help you to understand when or what you can hear. They will help you to understand when or what you may have trouble hearing.

EXERCISE 11

Read and answer each question. You may have to write a sentence to answer some questions. Everyone will have different answers to these questions. The answers are not in the Answer Key. Show your answers to your teacher.

1. What caused your hearing loss? (Ask your parents if you do not know. Read about the different causes on pages 13 and 14.)

2. How old were you when your parents found out about your hearing loss? (Ask your parents if you do not know.)

3. How old were you when you got your first hearing aid? (Ask your parents if you do not remember.)

4. What kind of hearing loss do you have? (Read pages 13 and 14 again if you do not know.)

    a. ____ conductive (There is a problem with my outer ear or middle ear.)

    b. ____ nerve (There is a problem with the nerves in my inner ear.)

    c. ____ mixed (There is a problem with my inner ear. There is also a problem with my outer or middle ear.)

5. Do your ears often feel clogged up?

   a. _____ yes   b. _____ no

6. Do you have fluid or tubes in your ears?

   a. _____ yes   b. _____ no   c. _____ I used to

7. Do you get many colds, sore throats, ear infections, or allergies that make your hearing seem worse?

   a. _____ yes   b. _____ no

8. Does anyone else in your family have a hearing loss?

   a. _____ yes (Who is it? _____)

   b. _____ no

9. How long will you have a hearing loss? (Read pages 13 and 14 again if you do not know.)

   a. _____ a short time (Why? _____)

   b. _____ a long time (Why? _____)

10. How long will you have to wear a hearing aid? (Read pages 13 and 14 again if you do not know.)

    a. _____ a short time (Why? _____)

    b. _____ a long time (Why? _____)

11. Where do you go to have your hearing tested? (Ask your parents if you do not know.)

    a. Write the name of the audiologist or audiology clinic.

    b. Write the address of the audiologist or audiology clinic location.

12. When was the last time your hearing was tested? Give the date. (Ask your parents if you do not remember.)

13. Has your hearing:

    a. _____ stayed the same?

    b. _____ gotten better?

    c. _____ gotten worse?

14. Do you hear noises inside your head all the time?

    a. _____ yes   b. _____ no

15. Do loud sounds hurt your ears?

    a. _____ yes   b. _____ no

16. Is it hard for you to tell where a sound is coming from?

    a. _____ yes   b. _____ no   c. _____ sometimes

17. Can you hear the doorbell ring or someone knocking at the door?

    a. _____ yes   b. _____ no   c. _____ sometimes

18. Can you hear the telephone ring?

    a. _____ yes   b. _____ no   c. _____ sometimes

19. Can you hear your own voice when you talk?

    a. _____ yes   b. _____ no   c. _____ sometimes

20. How do the voices of other people sound to you?

    a. _____ loud   b. _____ soft   c. _____ normal

21. Do you hear people's voices easily but still have a hard time understanding their words?

    a. _____ yes   b. _____ no   c. _____ sometimes

22. Can you understand people better if you watch their faces and lips when they talk?

    a. ____ yes   b. ____ no   c. ____ sometimes

23. Whom do you hear better?

    a. ____ men   b. ____ women   c. ____ they sound the same

24. Is it hard for you to hear when several people are talking at the same time?

    a. ____ yes   b. ____ no   c. ____ sometimes

25. Where do you hear better?

    a. ____ in a quiet place   b. ____ in a noisy place

26. When do you hear better?

    a. ____ when I am close to the person who is talking

    b. ____ when I am far away from the person who is talking

27. Do you tell all of your teachers that you have a hearing loss?

    a. ____ yes

    b. ____ no (Why not? _____)

28. Do any of your teachers give you extra help in school?

    a. ____ yes (Who? _____)

    b. ____ no (Do you wish they would? _____)

29. Do any of your teachers talk while writing on the chalkboard, which stops you from reading their lips?

    a. ____ yes (Who? _____)
        (Ask them to stop doing this!)

    b. ____ no

30. Do any of your teachers cover their faces with hands or books, which stops you from reading their lips?

    a. ____ yes (Who? _____)
        (Ask them to stop doing this!)

    b. ____ no

31. Do any of your teachers move around the room while teaching, which stops you from reading their lips?

    a. ____ yes (Who? _____)
       (Ask them to stop doing this!)

    b. ____ no

32. Do any of your teachers mumble when they talk, which makes it hard for you to hear them?

    a. ____ yes (Who? _____)
       (Ask them to stop doing this!)

    b. ____ no

33. Do all of your teachers write important things on the chalkboard so that you can read them?

    a. ____ yes

    b. ____ no (Who doesn't? _____)
       (Ask them to begin doing this!)

34. Do all of your teachers stand close to your desk when teaching so that you can hear them easily?

    a. ____ yes

    b. ____ no (Who doesn't? _____)
       (Ask them to begin doing this!)

35. Do all of your teachers repeat directions or assignments if you did not hear them?

    a. ____ yes

    b. ____ no (Who doesn't? _____)
       (Ask them to begin doing this!)

36. Are any of your classes noisy, which makes it hard for you to hear?

   a. _____ yes (Which ones? _____)

   b. _____ no

37. Do you have special classroom seating in all of your classes? (Read pages 17 and 18 again if you do not remember what special classroom seating means.)

   a. _____ yes

   b. _____ no (Which ones/why not? _____)
   (Ask the teacher to change your seat!)

38. Do you have a buddy in school who helps you when you do not hear something or takes notes during class for you?

   a. _____ yes (Who? _____)

   b. _____ no (Would you like one? _____)

39. Do you have trouble hearing the record player or cassette player in school?

   a. _____ yes   b. _____ no   c. _____ sometimes

40. Do you have trouble understanding films when you cannot see the speaker's face?

   a. _____ yes   b. _____ no   c. _____ sometimes

41. Do you have trouble hearing people talking over the loudspeaker in school?

   a. _____ yes   b. _____ no   c. _____ sometimes

42. Do you have trouble hearing what a teacher says during spoken tests, like a spelling test?

   a. _____ yes   b. _____ no   c. _____ sometimes

43. What special help do you need because of your hearing loss? Put a check in front of each correct answer. You may find up to six answers.

    With the help of my teachers, I must learn how to:

    a. _____ wear and care for a hearing aid.

    b. _____ listen better.

    c. _____ catch fish.

    d. _____ speechread better.

    e. _____ make good speech sounds.

    f. _____ dress myself.

    g. _____ put words together to make good sentences.

    h. _____ feed myself.

    i. _____ understand the meanings of many words.

44. How well do you hear the following things without a hearing aid? How well do you hear them with an aid? Write a few words about each one. Compare how you hear without the aid and with it.

How well do you hear:	*without your hearing aid*	*with your hearing aid*
a. over the phone?		
b. the TV?		
c. the radio?		
d. at the movies?		
e. in the classroom?		
f. in groups?		
g. at home?		

Lesson 6

How Do You Feel About Your Hearing Loss?

Many people have trouble hearing. Do you know anyone else who has a hearing loss? If you do not, you may feel alone. Maybe you would like to talk to someone about how it feels to have a hearing loss. Talking about your hearing problem can help you to feel better about it. You can talk to your teacher, your parents, or a friend about your hearing problem.

There are many questions about your hearing loss in this lesson. The answers to these questions are important. The answers will show how you feel about having a hearing problem.

After you answer the questions, you will read more about feelings. You will read about ways to feel better about your hearing loss.

Be honest when you answer these questions. Be honest about your feelings. Do not worry about giving the right answer. There are no right answers or wrong answers. Each person will have different answers.

EXERCISE 12

Read each question. Put a check in front of the best answer. You may have to write a sentence to answer some questions. Everyone will have different answers to these questions. The answers are not in the Answer Key. Show your answers to your teacher.

1. How do you feel about having a hearing loss?

    a. _____ I don't mind it.

    b. _____ I feel unhappy about it.

    c. _____ I feel angry about it.

    d. _____ Other: _____

2. Do you ever think, "Why did this happen to me?"

    a. _____ yes   b. _____ no

3. Do you want to hear better?

   a. _____ yes   b. _____ no

4. How do you think your parents feel about your hearing loss?

   a. _____ They don't mind it.

   b. _____ They feel unhappy about it.

   c. _____ They feel angry about it.

   d. _____ Other: _____

5. Do you have any brothers or sisters? If so, how do you think they feel about your hearing loss?

   a. _____ They don't mind it.

   b. _____ They feel unhappy about it.

   c. _____ They feel angry about it.

   d. _____ They tease me about it.

   e. _____ Other: _____

6. Does your family understand the problems you may have because of a hearing loss?

   a. _____ yes

   b. _____ no (What don't they understand? _____)

7. Besides your family, does anyone else know that you have a hearing loss?

   a. _____ yes (Who? _____)

   b. _____ no (Why not? _____)

8. Pretend someone asked you, "Do you have a hearing problem?" How would you feel?

   a. _____ I would not let it bother me.

   b. _____ I would feel angry about it.

c. _____ I would feel hurt or sad.

   d. _____ Other: _____

9. Pretend someone asked you, "Do you have a hearing problem?" What would you say?

   a. _____ I would say, "Yes, I do have trouble hearing."

   b. _____ I would say, "It is none of your business!"

   c. _____ I would say, "Why do you ask?"

   d. _____ I would not answer. I would change the subject and start talking about something else.

   e. _____ Other: _____

10. Are you ever afraid to tell people that you have trouble hearing?

    a. _____ yes (Who/when? _____)

    b. _____ no

11. Do you remind people that you have trouble hearing when they seem to forget?

    a. _____ yes (How? _____)

    b. _____ no

12. Does a hearing loss make you feel different from other people?

    a. _____ yes (How/when? _____)

    b. _____ no

13. Are you ever afraid to be with people because you may have trouble hearing them?

    a. _____ yes (Who/when? _____)

    b. _____ no

14. Would you rather be by yourself than with other people?

    a. _____ yes   b. _____ no

15. Do you stay away from people so that you do not have to talk to them?

   a. ____ yes (Who/when? _____)

   b. ____ no

16. Does a hearing loss ever stop you from talking to other people?

   a. ____ yes (Who/when? _____)

   b. ____ no

17. Do you think you have fewer friends because you cannot hear well?

   a. ____ yes (Why? _____)

   b. ____ no

18. Do people leave you out of conversations because you cannot keep up with them?

   a. ____ yes

   b. ____ no

19. Do you think people talk about you?

   a. ____ yes (Who/why? _____)

   b. ____ no

20. Does anyone ever make fun of your hearing problem?

   a. ____ yes (Who? _____)

   b. ____ no

21. Pretend someone teased you about your hearing problem. How would you feel?

   a. ____ I would not let it bother me.

   b. ____ I would feel angry about it.

   c. ____ I would feel hurt or sad.

   d. ____ Other: _____

22. Pretend someone teased you about your hearing problem. What would you do?

   a. _____ I would ignore it (do nothing).

   b. _____ I would fight back.

   c. _____ I would start to cry.

   d. _____ Other: _____

23. Does a hearing loss ever keep you from hearing what people say?

   a. _____ yes   b. _____ no

24. Do you ever feel angry when you do not hear what someone says?

   a. _____ yes   b. _____ no

25. Do you ever feel embarrassed when you do not hear someone?

   a. _____ yes   b. _____ no

26. Do you always ask someone to repeat a sentence if you did not hear it?

   a. _____ yes

   b. _____ no (Why not? _____)

27. When you do not hear what someone says, do you ever pretend that you heard it?

   a. _____ yes (Why? _____)

   b. _____ no

28. Do you ever pretend that you do not hear something at home, like your mother telling you to clean your room?

   a. _____ yes (What/when? _____)

   b. _____ no

29. Do you ever pretend that you do not hear something in school, like a homework assignment?

   a. _____ yes (What/when? _____)

   b. _____ no

30. Does a hearing loss ever make you feel dumb?

   a. _____ yes (When? _____)

   b. _____ no

31. Does a hearing problem ever stop you from doing what you would like to do?

   a. _____ yes (What/when? _____)

   b. _____ no

32. Are you ever embarrassed to sit in front or to get closer to the speaker so that you can hear better?

   a. _____ yes (When? _____)

   b. _____ no

33. Are you ever afraid to ask or answer questions in school because you may say the wrong thing?

   a. _____ yes   b. _____ no

34. Do you think you would get better grades in school if you did not have a hearing loss?

   a. _____ yes (Which subjects/why? _____)

   b. _____ no

35. Are you afraid that maybe you won't be able to go to college or get a certain job because of your hearing loss?

   a. _____ yes

   b. _____ no

   c. _____ I have not thought about it.

How to Feel Better About Your Hearing Loss

Nobody wants to have a hearing problem. But many people do have trouble hearing. You are one of them. You do have feelings about your hearing loss, too. All people have feelings about whatever problems they may have.

It is helpful to have good feelings about your hearing loss. How can you learn to feel better about it? Remember these things.

1. You are not alone! Many people have trouble hearing.
2. There is nothing wrong with having a hearing problem.
3. Tell yourself, "I do have a hearing loss. It is all right to have trouble hearing."
4. Tell other people that you have trouble hearing. Tell them what they can do to help you hear better.
5. Talking to other people is easier when they know about your hearing problem.
6. Nobody is perfect! Some people have trouble walking, seeing, learning, or talking. You happen to have trouble hearing.
7. You are not really different from other people. You are still a person. You are just like everybody else. You have the same wants, needs, feelings, and fears that all people have.
8. Be with people. Talk to them. Just be yourself. People will like you if you like yourself. People are not going to laugh at your hearing problem.
9. Just because you miss a few words, do not think that people are talking about you.
10. When you do not hear what someone says, never pretend that you heard. This could get you into trouble. You may be saying yes without knowing it!
11. When you do not hear what someone says, ask the person to say it again. This shows you are really trying to listen. It shows that you want to hear what is being said.
12. Do not pretend that you didn't hear what someone said when you really did. This may get you out of doing things. But you are not being honest when you pretend to miss something. If you do this all the time, it may mean that you are lazy.
13. Do not say, "I can't do that because of my hearing problem." Don't let a hearing loss stop you from doing something that you want to do. Try it! You may be good at it. You can do everything (or almost everything) that other people do.
14. You do not have a hearing loss because you are a "bad" person. You did not do anything wrong. You did not cause it.
15. Do not blame your parents for your hearing problem. They do not want you to have trouble hearing. It is not their fault.
16. Your parents love you very much. They love you even though you have trouble hearing. It does not matter to them that you have a hearing problem.
17. Having a hearing problem is nobody's fault.
18. You will have mixed feelings about your hearing loss. Sometimes you may feel angry, embarrassed, sad, or dumb. Don't worry about having these feelings. It is natural to feel all of them. These feelings will last for only a short time. Then they will go away and you will feel better.

PART II

All About Hearing Aids

Lesson 7

How a Hearing Aid Helps You

A hearing aid helps you to hear many different sounds during the day. That is why you should wear your hearing aid every day, all day long! You should wear it from the time you wake up until you go to bed again. The aid cannot help you to hear better if it is inside your desk or pocket.

EXERCISE 13

Your aid helps you to hear some important sounds. You may hear these sounds in school, at home, or when you go out of your house. Look at the list below. Read each sentence. Write **S** in front of the sentence if it describes a sound you hear in school. Write **H** in front of the sentence if it describes a sound you hear at home. Write **O** if you hear the sound when you go out of your house. You may go out of your house to eat, shop, visit, or to go to religious services, parties, and movies.

You can hear some of the sounds in more than one place. You may write two or three letters if you can hear the sound in different places.

Check your answers with the Answer Key when you are finished.

1. A hearing aid helps me to:

   a. _____ hear what the principal and my teachers say.

   b. _____ hear what my friends say.

   c. _____ hear sounds from car horns, trains, trucks, fire engines, ambulances, a police officer's whistle, motorboats, and birds singing.

   d. _____ hear the television, radio, and stereo.

   e. _____ hear what my classmates say.

   f. _____ hear at the movies.

   g. _____ hear what my mother, father, sisters, or brothers say.

   h. _____ hear what visitors and neighbors say.

   i. _____ hear what people say in stores and restaurants or in large meetings.

j. ____ hear and improve my own speech (make it better).

k. ____ hear different sounds like a bell ringing, students walking in the hallway, doors closing, people knocking at doors, and people talking over the loudspeaker.

l. ____ hear what club leaders or Scout Leaders say.

m. ____ hear films, the record player, cassette player, or tape recorder.

n. ____ hear and understand rules for games.

o. ____ hear sounds from an alarm clock, a vacuum cleaner, a doorbell, a telephone, a smoke alarm, a lawnmower, someone hammering, dishes rattling, and water running.

p. ____ hear the bus driver.

q. ____ hear the sounds my pets make.

r. ____ hear traffic when I cross the street.

s. ____ hear music, talking, and laughing.

t. ____ hear what people say on the bus, at parties, and at clubs.

2. Do you wear your hearing aid every day? How many hours do you wear it each day? Where do you usually wear the aid? Let's find out by filling in this chart.

Look at the chart on the next page. Write the date in the left column. Write in how many hours you wore the aid on that date. If you wore the aid at home, write a little note telling when (for dinner, for company, for listening to the radio, etc.). Write how much you wore the aid in school (all morning, for English, for reading, etc.). Then write whether you wore the aid for any outside activities (for going to a movie, for eating at a restaurant, for roller-skating, etc.).

The first line is done so you can see how to do the chart. Fill in the chart until each line is used. Show the chart to your teacher each time you fill in a line.

Remember: You should wear your hearing aid every day, all day!

Hearing Aid Use

Date	How Many Hours	Where		
		Home	School	Outside Activities
March 22	11	for TV	all day	for Scouts

Lesson 8

Hearing Aids

New Vocabulary

You will learn these words as you read this lesson. Say each word. Read its definition.

Air receiver: sends sounds from a body aid into the earmold.

Battery: the power source for a hearing aid.

Battery holder: the area where the battery fits inside an aid.

Behind-the-ear aid: a hearing aid worn behind a person's ear.

Body aid: a hearing aid that is worn near a person's chest.

Bone receiver: sends sounds from the aid into the bones of the head. It fits behind the ear. It moves back and forth.

Case: the outside covering of a hearing aid. It protects the wires and tiny parts inside the aid.

Clip: the part that holds a body aid onto a person's shirt.

Cord: a wire that carries sound.

Cross-over aid: a hearing aid that sends sound from one ear to the other ear.

Earmold: sends sounds from the aid into the outer ear. It fits into the ear.

Eyeglass aid: a hearing aid built into a pair of eyeglasses.

Frames: the part of an eyeglass aid that holds the aid near the ear.

Headband: holds a bone receiver on the bone behind the ear.

Hook: carries sound from the aid to the tube. It fits over the ear.

In-the-ear aid: a hearing aid worn inside the outer ear.

Jacket (or harness): a special pocket that holds a body aid near a person's chest.

Microphone: pulls sound into the hearing aid.

Microphone and telephone control: makes the microphone control and the telephone control work at the same time. It helps a person hear other sounds in the room while talking on the telephone. It can help a person hear sounds through special wires stretched around a room.

On-off control: turns a hearing aid on and off.

Screws: the parts that hold the case together on some hearing aids.

Telephone control: helps a person hear better over the telephone.

Tone control: makes some sounds louder than other sounds.

Tube: carries sound from the hook to the earmold.

Volume control: makes the sounds from a hearing aid loud or soft.

What Do Hearing Aids Do?

Everyone does not wear the same kind of hearing aid. Different people wear different hearing aids. All hearing aids do the same thing, even though they may look different. All hearing aids make sound louder so that you can hear it.

You will read about different types of hearing aids. You will read about how they work. You will read about the many parts hearing aids can have.

Hearing Aids with an Earmold

Most, but not all, people wear a hearing aid that has an **earmold.** An earmold fits into the outer ear. It sends sound waves from the aid into the outer ear. Sound waves hit against the eardrum and make it move. This makes the three tiny bones move. Then the nerves inside the cochlea move. That is how a person hears with an aid that has an earmold.

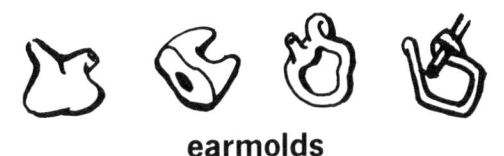

earmolds

Hearing Aids with a Bone Receiver

All hearing aids do not have an earmold. Some people cannot wear an earmold in their ear. A person can be born without an outer ear. A person can have a hole in one or both eardrums. Maybe the person always has fluid in the middle ear. These people wear a hearing aid without an earmold. The aid has a **bone receiver** instead of an earmold.

The bone receiver is held on the bone behind the ear. It sends sound waves from the aid into the inner ear. The bone receiver moves back and forth. You can see it move. You can feel it move. It makes the bones of the head move. Then the nerve endings inside the cochlea move. That is how a person hears with an aid that has a bone receiver.

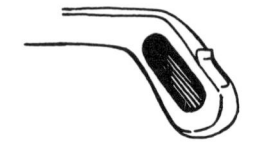

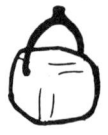

bone receivers

EXERCISE 14

Can you answer these questions about hearing aids? Check your answers with the Answer Key when you are finished.

1. Write T if the sentence is true. Write F if the sentence is false.

    a. _____ Everyone can wear the same kind of hearing aid.

    b. _____ All hearing aids have an earmold.

    c. _____ Everyone can wear an earmold in the outer ear.

    d. _____ Some hearing aids have a bone receiver instead of an earmold.

    e. _____ The only thing a hearing aid does is make sound louder.

    f. _____ An earmold fits into the inner ear.

    g. _____ A bone receiver helps people to hear by moving the bones of the head.

    h. _____ A bone receiver is held on the bones of a person's foot.

    i. _____ An earmold sends sound waves into the outer ear.

    j. _____ A bone receiver sends sound waves into the middle ear.

2. Does your hearing aid have a bone receiver?

    a. ____ yes   b. ____ no

3. Does your hearing aid have an earmold?

    a. ____ yes   b. ____ no

Different Kinds of Aids

Now you will read about five kinds of hearing aids—body aids, behind-the-ear aids, in-the-ear aids, eyeglass aids, and cross-over aids.

Body Aids

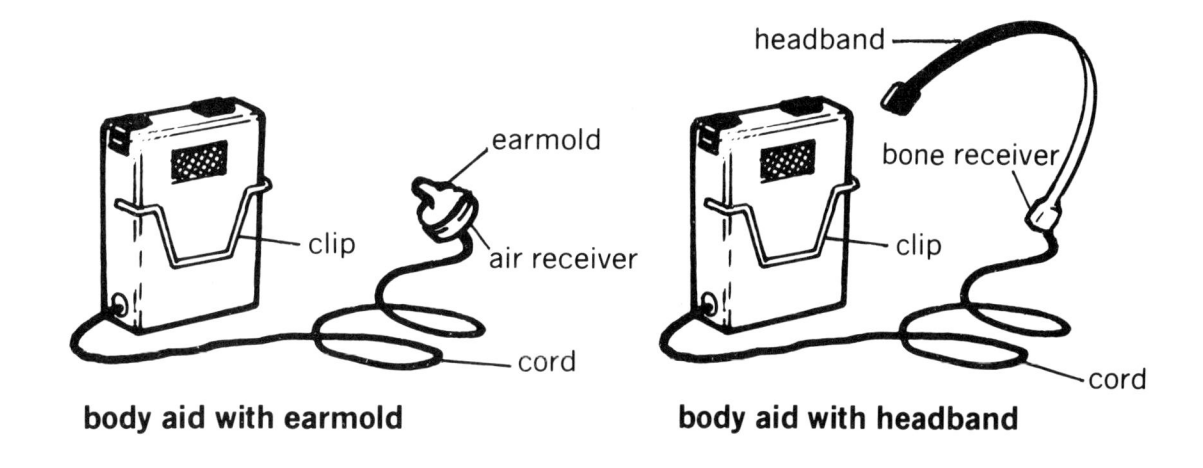

body aid with earmold   body aid with headband

A **body aid** is worn on the chest. A **clip** holds the aid onto a shirt. A **jacket** (some people call it a **harness**) holds the aid near the chest if the shirt has no pocket.

A body aid has a **cord.** A cord is a wire. It carries sound from the hearing aid to a receiver.

An **air receiver** looks like a button. It sends sound waves into an **earmold.** An earmold fits into the outer ear. It sends sound waves into the ear. A **bone receiver** sends sound waves into the head. Sounds make the bone receiver move back and forth. This makes the bones of the head move. A **headband** goes on the head. It holds a bone receiver on the bone behind the ear.

Behind-the-Ear Aids

A **behind-the-ear aid** is worn behind the ear. The aid is held on the ear by a short **hook.** The hook carries sound from the aid to a **tube.** The tube carries sound waves from the hook to the earmold.

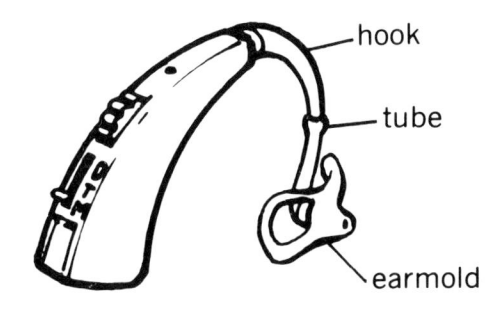

behind-the-ear aid

In-the-Ear Aids

An **in-the-ear aid** is very small. The whole hearing aid fits inside the outer ear. Many in-the-ear aids are built into an earmold. All the parts are inside the earmold. Some in-the-ear aids do not have a whole earmold.

An in-the-ear aid has no hook, tube, or cord. Sound goes into a tiny opening called a **microphone.** The sound waves become louder as they travel through the different parts inside the aid. Then the earmold sends the sound waves into the ear.

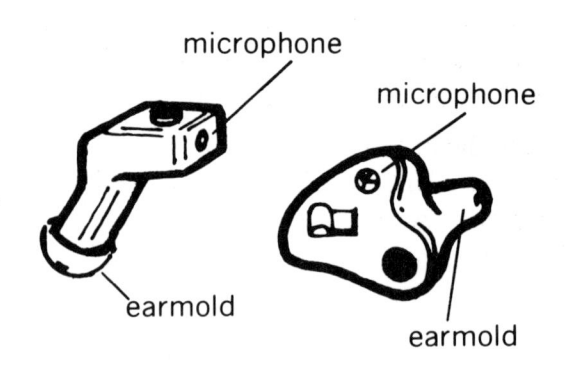

in-the-ear aids

Eyeglass Aids

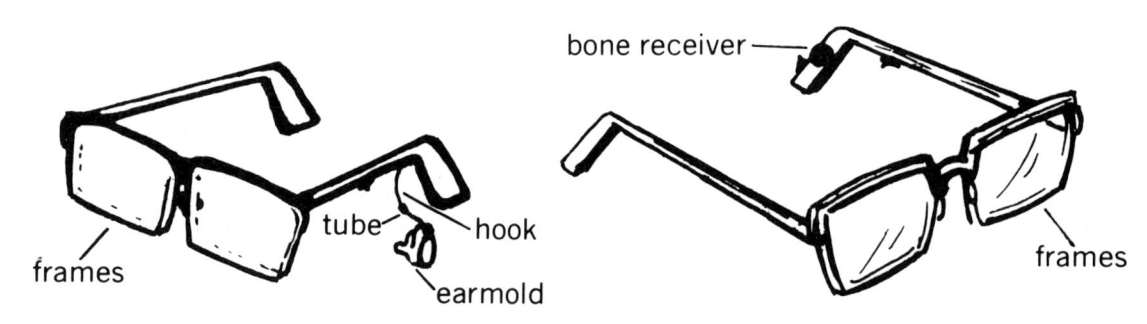

eyeglass aid with earmold

eyeglass aid with bone receiver

A hearing aid can be part of a pair of glasses. This kind of hearing aid is called an **eyeglass aid.** The hearing aid is built into the **frames.**

The frames of the glasses hold the hearing aid near the ear. A hook and tube may carry sound from the aid to an earmold. Or, the frames may hold a bone receiver on the bone behind the ear.

An eyeglass aid helps people who wear glasses and a hearing aid, too. But many people who wear glasses and an aid do not wear an eyeglass aid. How can they do this if they do not have an eyeglass aid? It's easy—their glasses fit over or under their hearing aid without much trouble. At first it may feel strange, but that does not last long. People get used to it quickly. It is easy to wear a hearing aid and glasses at the same time.

Cross-over Aids

In some hearing aids, the sound crosses over from one ear to the other. This lets a person hear from both sides of the head at the same time. A **cross-over aid** is really two hearing aids. There is an aid on each ear.

The hearing aids can be worn behind the ear. Or, the aids can be built into a pair of glasses. Many people wear two behind-the-ear aids with a cord between them. The cord goes behind the neck and under the hair. An eyeglass aid has two hearing aids built into the frames. The frames hold the aids near the ear.

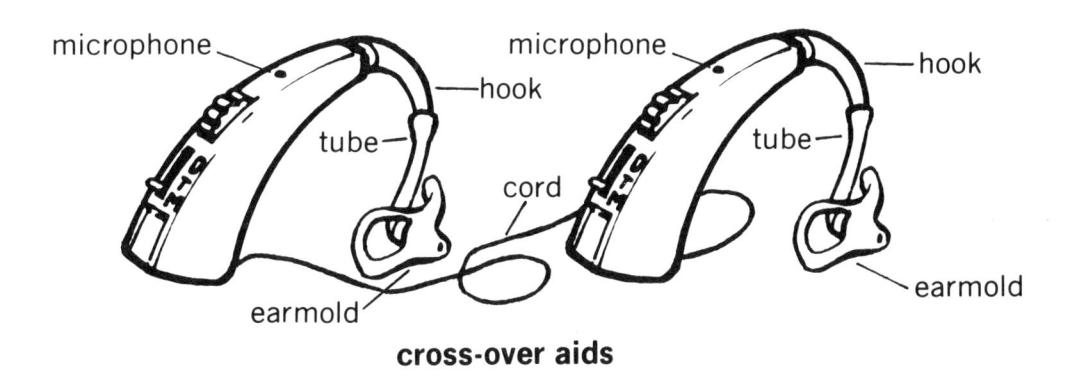

cross-over aids

Here is how a cross-over aid works: Sound goes into a microphone on one of the aids. The sound quickly travels to the other aid and into the other ear. The sound waves may move through the air. Or, they may move through a cord. The cord carries sound from one aid to the other. In an eyeglass aid, the cord is inside the frames. You cannot see the cord.

EXERCISE 15

You have read much about different kinds of hearing aids. Answer these questions about your hearing aid. Everyone will have different answers to these questions. The answers are not in the Answer Key. Show your answers to your teacher.

1. Which kind of hearing aid do you wear?

    a. ____ body aid

    b. ____ behind-the-ear aid

    c. ____ in-the-ear aid

    d. ____ eyeglass aid

    e. ____ cross-over aid

2. How many hearing aids do you wear?

   a. ____ one   b. ____ two

3. In which ear do you wear a hearing aid?

   a. ____ right ear   b. ____ left ear   c. ____ both ears

4. Did someone show you how to use the aid when you first got it?

   a. ____ yes (Who? _____)

   b. ____ no

5. Did someone show you how to take care of the aid when you first got it?

   a. ____ yes (Who? _____)

   b. ____ no

6. Can you put on your hearing aid without help from anyone?

   a. ____ yes

   b. ____ no (Who helps you? _____)

Other Hearing Aid Parts

Battery and Battery Holder

All hearing aids need power to work. Most aids get power to work from a **battery.** The **battery holder** keeps the battery inside the aid.

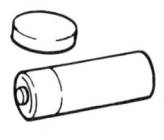

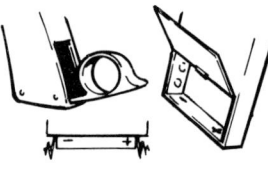

batteries   **battery holders**

A few hearing aids do not need a battery to work. They get power to work from a special box. This special box comes with the hearing aid. The aid stays in the box every night while the person is sleeping. This box gives the aid enough power to work the next day.

Case and Screws

The **case** is the outside covering of an aid. It covers the wires and tiny parts inside the aid. The case keeps the wires and tiny parts from getting dirty or lost.

Tiny **screws** may hold the case together, so the parts inside the case will not fall out. Some cases are held together with a special glue.

cases

screws

Microphone

Sounds from the air go into a **microphone.** The microphone pulls sound into the hearing aid. Then the aid makes the sound louder before sending the sound into your ear.

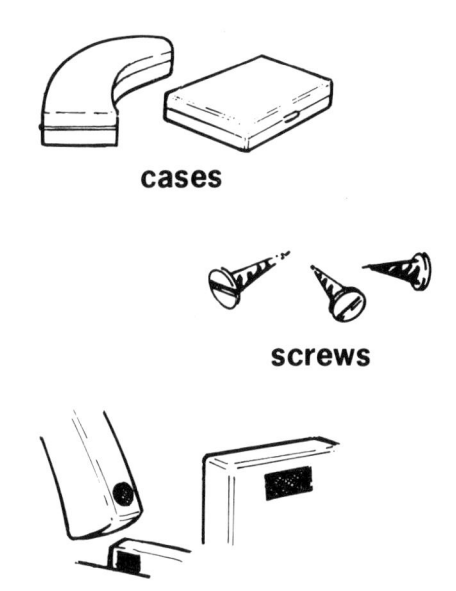

microphones

Controls

Hearing aids have different **controls.** Controls make the aid do different things.

1. *On-off control:* turns the aid on and off. When the aid is turned off, the microphone does not work. The letter *O* usually means the aid is turned off. When the aid is turned on, the microphone works. The letter *M* usually means the microphone is turned on. The letter *S* usually means the microphone will block out louder, noisy sounds. This helps you to hear softer sounds more easily.

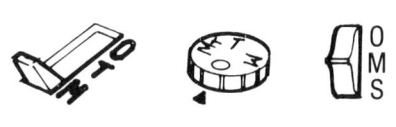

on-off controls

2. *Volume control:* makes sounds louder or softer. You can make the aid sound louder or softer by moving the volume control.

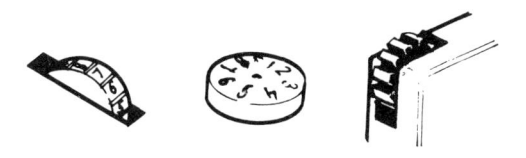

volume controls

3. *Tone control:* makes some sounds louder than other sounds. It can make low sounds (like a drum) louder. It can make high sounds (like a whistle) louder. The tone control has different letters on it. The letter *L* means low sounds are being made louder by the aid. *H* means high sounds are being made louder than other sounds. *N* means that no sounds are louder than others. All low, middle, and high sounds have the same loudness. Not all hearing aids have a tone control.

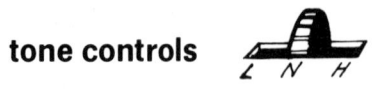

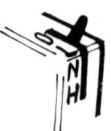

tone controls

4. *Telephone control:* some people have trouble hearing over the telephone. That is why some aids have a telephone control. A telephone control helps people hear better over the telephone. The letter *T* means telephone. When the telephone control is turned on, the aid picks up sounds from the telephone. Sounds from the telephone are made louder. Sounds in the room around the person are not made louder. This helps a person to use the telephone more easily.

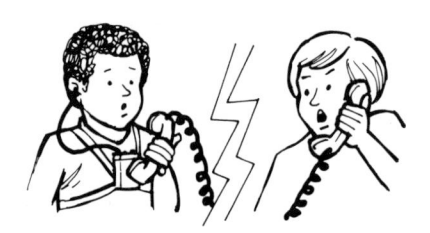

**how to use the telephone
with a hearing aid**

A telephone control is easy to use. Turn the telephone control to *T.* Hold the listening end of the telephone against the case of your aid. If you have a body aid, hold the phone's listening end near your chest, close to the microphone. For all other aids, hold the listening end near your ear so that the sounds go into the microphone. Move the phone around to find the place where the voice sounds loudest. (You can add special equipment to your telephone that will make the caller's voice louder. This equipment, called an amplifier, is available from your telephone company or hearing aid dealer.)

You must turn off the telephone control when you hang up the phone. You won't hear sounds in the room around you if you leave it on. Change the control so that the microphone is turned on.

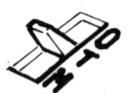

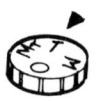

telephone control

5. *Microphone and telephone control:* makes the microphone control and the telephone control work at the same time. The letters *MT* or *B* usually mean the microphone and telephone control is turned on. The *MT* or *B* control does two things.

   a. It helps you hear voices over the telephone. You can hear your own voice when you talk. You can hear sounds in the room around you, too.
   b. It helps you hear sounds through a special set of wires. The wires are stretched around a room. The room may be a classroom for students with hearing problems. Or, the wires can be stretched around someone's living room. The wires lead to a teacher's microphone, a television, a radio, or a stereo. The wires make sounds and voices louder. They are easier to hear. You can hear your own voice when you talk. You can hear sounds in the room around you, too.

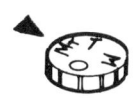

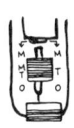

microphone and telephone controls

EXERCISE 16

You have read much about different hearing aid parts. Can you answer these questions about your hearing aid? Put a check in front of the correct answers. Everyone will have different answers to these questions. The answers are not in the Answer Key. Show your answers to your teacher.

1. Does your hearing aid get power to work from batteries?

   a. ____ Yes, my hearing aid uses batteries.

   b. ____ No, my aid gets power to work from a special box.

2. Do you know how to turn the aid on and off?

   a. ____ yes (Can you do it while you are wearing the aid? _____)

   b. ____ no (Ask someone to show you!)

3. Do you know how to change the volume control (make the aid sound louder or softer)?

   a. ____ yes (Can you do it while you are wearing the aid? _____)

   b. ____ no (Ask someone to show you!)

4. Do you have trouble hearing over the telephone?

   a. ____ yes   b. ____ no

5. Does your aid have a telephone control?

   a. ____ yes (Do you use it? _____)

   (Can you turn it on while you are wearing the aid? _____)

   b. ____ no (Do you wish it did? _____)

6. Does your aid have a tone control?

   a. ____ yes (Do you use it? _____)

   (Can you turn it on while you are wearing the aid? _____)

   b. ____ no

7. Does your aid have a microphone and telephone control together (*MT* or *B*)?

   a. ____ yes (Do you use it? _____)

   (Can you turn it on while you are wearing the aid? _____)

   b. ____ no

EXERCISE 17

Hearing aids can have many different parts. You have already read about them. The different parts are listed below. Your hearing aid will not have each one. Draw a line through any part your aid does not have.

Find the parts that belong to your hearing aid. Write a sentence telling what each part does. Check your answers with the Answer Key when you are finished.

1. Battery: _____

_____

2. Battery holder: _____

_____

3. Case: _____

_____

4. Screws: _____
   _____

5. Microphone: _____
   _____

6. On-off control: _____
   _____

7. Volume control: _____
   _____

8. Tone control: _____
   _____

9. Telephone control: _____
   _____

10. Microphone and telephone control: _____
    _____

11. Hook: _____
    _____

12. Tube: _____
    _____

13. Cord: _____
    _____

14. Earmold: _____
    _____

15. Air receiver: _____
    _____

16. Bone receiver: _____
    _____

17. Clip: _____
    _____

18. Jacket: _____
    _____

19. Headband: _____
    _____

20. Frames: _____
    _____

EXERCISE 18

Look at your hearing aid. Draw a picture of your aid below. Be sure to draw all the parts of your aid. See if you can name each part as you draw it. Don't forget to draw the battery, too! Put the number of your battery on the picture of the battery.

Look at the picture you drew. Now draw an arrow pointing to each part of your aid. Don't forget any parts! Write the name of each part next to the arrows. Everyone's picture will look different. The Answer Key does not have pictures of hearing aids. Show your picture to your teacher.

Lesson 9

Hearing Aid Check

You need your hearing aid so you can hear better. The aid cannot help you if it is not working well. It cannot help you if you are not wearing it, either.

Check your aid each day to make sure it is working well. It takes less than one minute. It is easy to do. Follow these directions:

1. *Look at the aid before putting it on.* Look at each part of the aid. Is each part clean? Is each part dry? Is anything broken? Is anything loose?
2. *Listen to how the aid sounds.* Put on your hearing aid. Turn on the microphone. Move the volume control so that sounds get louder and softer. Listen to the aid as you move the volume control. If your aid has a cord, move it back and forth between your fingers. Listen to the aid as you move the cord.

   Does the aid sound strong or weak? Does it buzz? Does it whistle? Does it go off and on? Is it dead? Is it scratchy? All of these things mean something is wrong with your aid. You must fix the problem before the aid will work well again. Look at Lesson 18, "Fixing Hearing Aid Problems." It will help you find the problem with your aid.

EXERCISE 19

How does your hearing aid look and sound today? Let's find out. Turn to the next page. You will see a chart. This chart will help you to check your aid. Check your hearing aid right now!

Put a checkmark (√) under each part that looks good and works well. Put an X under any part that does not look good or work well. Skip the parts your aid does not have. Fix any problems with your aid. Write what you did to the aid. An example is given to help you.

Fill in the chart every day until each line is used. Show the chart to your teacher each time you fill in a line.

Hearing Aid Check

Date	battery & holder	case/screws	controls	microphone	hook & tube	cord/plugs	earmold	air/bone receiver	jacket/clip	headband or frames	Remarks
Sept. 19	x	✓	✓	✓	✓						Changed battery

Lesson 10

Important Hearing Aid Information

New Vocabulary

You will learn these words as you read this lesson. Say each word. Read its definition.

Battery number: the number on a battery. This number tells the size of the battery.

Cord length: how long a hearing aid cord is.

Cord type: the kind of cord that fits on a hearing aid.

Hearing aid dealer: a person who sells and fixes hearing aids.

Make: the name of the company that makes the hearing aid.

Model: the second name, letters, or numbers printed on the aid. It gives more information about the hearing aid.

Serial number: a special number given to a hearing aid. Each hearing aid has a different serial number.

What You Should Know

You should know all about your hearing aid. This information is important. It tells you many things about your hearing aid.

This information helps you or your parents in many ways. It helps you to find the aid if it gets lost or stolen. It helps you to know the difference between your aid and others that look like yours. It helps you to get the aid fixed. It helps you to buy a new battery or cord for the aid.

Here is the information you should know about your aid.

1. the make
2. the model
3. the serial number
4. the battery number
5. the cord type
6. the cord length
7. the name, address, and telephone number of your hearing aid dealer, audiologist, or audiology clinic

The Make

The **make** is the name of the company that makes your aid. The name is often printed on the case of the aid. A few companies that make aids are Zenith, Phonic Ear, Sonotone, Danavox, and Radioear. Look at your hearing aid case. Find the make of your hearing aid.

The Model

Sometimes an aid has a second name. The second name is called the **model**. Sometimes the model is made up of letters or numbers. The model gives more information about the kind of aid you have. It is often printed on the case. Here are examples of different models—Emblem, Sentry, A770 Gold, HC-527, 980, 670-S, and PE-1. Look at your hearing aid case. Find the model of your hearing aid.

The Serial Number

The **serial number** is the special number of your hearing aid. The serial number is often printed on the case. Sometimes it is printed inside the battery holder. No one else has the same serial number as you do. This is how you can tell your aid from someone else's, even if the two aids look alike. Here are examples of different serial numbers—2128749, 76-8361, and GFE-29. Can you find the serial number on your hearing aid?

The Battery Number

The **battery number** is printed on the battery. It tells what size battery your aid uses. There are many sizes of batteries, but only one size fits your aid. Only one size battery makes your aid work right. Here are examples of different battery numbers—AA, 933, 675, 312, 76, and 13. What battery number does your hearing aid use?

The Cord Type

Does your aid have a cord? If so, be careful when buying a new one. All cords are not the same. You must buy the right kind of cord for your aid. If you don't, the aid will not work right. To find the **cord type**, look in the book that came with your aid. The book tells you which kind of cord to buy. Some cords have two "teeth" on their plugs. Some cords have three "teeth." Here are examples of different cord types—96644, 600:61, TW, and TD-AD. What cord type does your aid use?

The Cord Length

Cords come in different lengths, too. Some cords are short. They may be 12 or 18 inches long. Some cords are longer. They can be 30 or 40 inches long. The **cord length** is important. A cord that is too long for you will get knots in it. A cord that is too short will keep pulling out of the case. How long is your cord? Get a ruler. Measure the length of your cord right now!

Your Hearing Aid Dealer

A **hearing aid dealer** is a person who sells and fixes hearing aids. An audiologist or audiology clinic may sell and fix hearing aids, too. Where did you buy your hearing aid? That is where you must take the aid if it breaks. Find out the name of your hearing aid dealer, audiologist, or clinic. Find out the telephone number. Then you can call if you have a question about the aid. You should also know the address of your hearing aid dealer, audiologist, or clinic. Then you will know where to take the aid when it needs to be fixed.

EXERCISE 20

You have read much about important hearing aid information. See if you can answer these questions. Check your answers with the Answer Key when you are finished.

1. What number makes a hearing aid different from any other hearing aid? Find one answer.

    a. ____ the model number

    b. ____ the serial number

    c. ____ the battery number

2. What number tells which battery an aid uses? Find one answer.

    a. ____ the model number

    b. ____ the serial number

    c. ____ the battery number

3. What does the *make* of a hearing aid mean? Find one answer.

    The make is:

    a. ____ the year the hearing aid was made

    b. ____ where the hearing aid was made

    c. ____ the name of the company that made the hearing aid

4. The *model* gives more information about a hearing aid. Read the sentences below. Which ones are not true about the model? Find four answers.

   a. _____ It tells what color the aid is.

   b. _____ It can be a second name for the aid.

   c. _____ It can be letters or numbers.

   d. _____ It can be printed on the earmold.

   e. _____ It can be printed on the case.

   f. _____ It tells how old the aid is.

   g. _____ It tells how much the aid costs.

5. What does a hearing aid dealer do? Find two answers.

   A hearing aid dealer:

   a. _____ breaks aids.

   b. _____ sells aids.

   c. _____ paints aids.

   d. _____ makes aids.

   e. _____ fixes aids.

6. John needs a new cord for his aid. He goes into a store to buy one. What must he know about the cord? Find two answers.

   a. _____ the length of the cord

   b. _____ the weight of the cord

   c. _____ the serial number of the cord

   d. _____ the type of the cord

   e. _____ the battery number of the hearing aid

7. It is important to buy the right kind of battery or cord for your aid. What will happen if you do not? Find one answer.

   a. _____ The aid will get very hot.

b. _____ The aid will begin to smoke.

c. _____ The aid will catch on fire.

d. _____ The aid will break into many pieces.

e. _____ The aid will not work right.

8. Here is a place to write down the important information about your hearing aid. Someday you may need to know this information. Then you can just look on this page. It will be easy for you to find the information. Be sure to change the information if you get a new hearing aid. Show this information to your teacher.

Hearing aid:

    Make _____

    Model _____

    Serial number _____

    Battery number _____

    Cord type and length _____

Hearing aid dealer, audiologist, or audiology clinic:

    Name _____

    Telephone number _____

    Address _____

    _____

Lesson 11

Questions People Ask About Hearing Aids

People who wear hearing aids have many questions about them. You may have some questions about your hearing aid.

Here are the questions that people often ask. Each question is answered. The questions and their answers are important. They help you to learn more about your hearing aid. They help you to learn more about your hearing loss.

Read each question and its answer. Do you see any of your own questions here?

What does a hearing aid do?

A hearing aid does only one thing: It makes sounds louder. It helps a person to hear sounds by making them louder. It helps a person to hear more sounds. It helps a person to hear better.

Why do I need a hearing aid?

You need an aid because you have a hearing loss. Sound must be made louder before you can hear it. A hearing aid makes sound louder for you. It makes sound loud enough for you to hear. A hearing aid helps you to hear better.

Why am I wearing this hearing aid?

There are many different hearing aids to choose from. Your audiologist chose a certain aid for you. You are wearing a certain aid because it helps you more than the other aids. Your aid helps you to hear softer sounds, hear softer noises, hear softer speech, and understand speech better.

Does an aid cure my hearing loss?

A hearing aid helps you to hear better. That is all it does. An aid does not take away your hearing loss. It does not cure your hearing problem. You still have a hearing loss.

You do not hear the same as other people even while you are wearing an aid. Hearing with an aid is not the same as hearing with your ears. Sound is changed as it goes through a hearing aid. What you hear with an aid is different from what other people hear.

How can I get used to the aid?

There is more to wearing an aid than just putting it on. It takes time to get used to a hearing aid. You must get used to how the aid feels. You must get used to how the aid sounds.

Be patient. Do not give up easily. Wearing an aid takes much practice. It may take a few weeks or months to get used to wearing the aid. It is helpful if you want to hear better. You must want to wear the aid. The aid cannot help you if you are not wearing it.

Follow these steps for learning how to use your hearing aid.

1. Learn the different parts of your aid. Name them. Know what each part does. Learn how to put in the battery.
2. Practice putting on the aid. Sit in front of a mirror. Use both hands. Ask someone to help you. After a while you will not need to look in a mirror. You will not need anyone to help you.
3. Learn how to use all the controls while wearing the aid. Change the controls without looking. Know how to turn the aid on and off. Know how to change the volume control. Know how to change the other controls.
4. Wear the aid around your house at first. Start by wearing it for a short time. Wear the aid for a longer time each day. Do this until you are wearing the aid all day.
5. Start with a low volume. Turn the volume a little higher each day. Do this until louder sounds do not bother you. Do this until the volume is as loud as the audiologist says it should be.
6. Wear the aid in quiet places at first. Then try it in noisier places. Do this until the noise does not bother you.
7. Wear the aid around one or two people at first. Get used to listening to them talk. Then try wearing the aid when several people are together.
8. Wear the aid in school. Start by wearing it for the most important subjects. Or, wear it for a few hours each day. Do this until you are wearing the aid all day in school.
9. Start wearing the aid when you go places. Try it in a store. Try it at the movies. Try it when you are eating in a restaurant. Try it every place where there are sounds to hear.

When does an aid help me the most?

A hearing aid helps you to hear best when

1. It is quiet—noise can make listening hard to do.
2. You are close to the speaker—the speaker's voice will be louder.
3. The aid is working well—take good care of your aid.

Why does my voice sound louder than other people's?

An aid helps you to hear your own voice. It helps you to use better speech sounds when you talk.

You are close to the microphone of your hearing aid. Your voice goes into the microphone when you talk. The aid makes your voice louder. The sound of your voice goes into your ear. You can hear what you are saying. Your voice sounds louder than someone else's because you are closer to the microphone. Your voice goes into the microphone first.

Why do people tell me to talk louder?

Many people who wear a hearing aid speak very softly. Do you think your voice is loud enough when you talk? Does it sound loud to you? That's because you are close to the microphone.

Talk louder when other people say they cannot hear you. Your voice is not as loud as you think it is. It may sound loud enough to you. But it is not loud enough for others to hear easily.

Why is the hearing aid so noisy?

A hearing aid makes all sounds louder. It makes nice sounds, like birds singing, louder. It makes people's voices louder so you can hear what they are saying. A hearing aid also makes noise louder. Noisy sounds, like car horns and people coughing, become louder.

Any sound that goes into the microphone is made louder by the aid. The hearing aid will sound noisy if there is much noise around you.

What can I do about the noise I hear?

You may not want to hear the noise that an aid makes louder. The noise may make you feel nervous. It may make you feel tired.

Noise can make listening harder to do. It may keep you from hearing important sounds. It may keep you from hearing what a person says.

You must block out the noise you do not want to hear. A good listener hears important sounds like a voice or a telephone ringing. A good listener does not listen to noise made by coughing or chairs scraping on the floor.

Do not try to listen to many sounds at the same time. Pick out the most important sound. Listen to that sound. Try not to hear all the other sounds.

Learning to block out noise takes practice. Be patient. Practice listening to important sounds. Try not to hear noisy sounds.

How can my eyes help me?

Use your eyes! They help you to understand what people are saying. Your eyes and ears make a good team when you use them together.

You must watch a speaker carefully. Look at these things when a person is talking.
1. *The face*—Is the speaker happy, sad, angry, bored, or confused? Is the speaker smiling or frowning? Is the speaker looking at you or at someone else?
2. *The mouth*—Are the speaker's lips open, closed, or rounded? Are the teeth open or closed? Is the tongue tip up, down, or between the teeth?
3. *The hands and body*—Is the speaker pointing at you or at something else? Does the speaker's head nod yes or no?

Watching all of these things is called **speechreading**. Speechreading is not just watching a person's lips. It is also watching the speaker's face, hands, and body. It means watching the whole person.

Watching all of these things is important. They help you to know what a person is saying. They help you to know how a person feels. Your eyes can be very helpful. Use them all the time! Use them with your hearing.

Why is it hard to listen in a group of people?

It is hard to listen when many people are together. There can be a lot of noise. Everyone may be talking at the same time. All the voices can confuse you. You may not understand what anyone is saying.

What can you do to hear better? Listen to only one person at a time. Stay close to that person. This will make the person's voice louder and easier to hear. Try to block out other voices and noises. Watch the person's face and mouth. Watch the person's hand and body movements, too. This can help you to understand what the person is saying.

Does a hearing aid make speech clearer?

Do you have a nerve loss? If you do, then you may not hear parts of words. Your ears may hear some sounds, but not all sounds. You may hear someone's voice easily, but not understand what is being said. For example, when someone says, "It is my birthday," you may not hear every speech sound. You may only hear, "I__ i__ __y __ir_____ay."

Speech may not sound clear to you. It may sound fuzzy. It may seem like people always mumble. Do you have this problem? If so, a hearing aid will not make speech clearer. The aid will make speech louder, but not clearer.

You may not hear every word the speaker says. What can you do about this problem? You can do several things.
1. Watch the speaker closely. Speechreading can help you to understand many of the words.
2. Fill in the sounds or words you missed by thinking about what the speaker is saying. Do not spend time worrying about words you missed! It is better to think about what the speaker is going to say next.

3. Get the general idea of what was said. Do not try to hear every single word the speaker says. Just try to get the general idea of what is being said. You may understand what the speaker said, even though you did not hear every word.

What should I do when I don't understand someone?

Ask the speaker to repeat what was said if you did not hear it. Don't worry, the speaker will not be angry. The person will be glad that you are asking a question. This shows that you really want to hear what the person is saying. It shows that you are really trying to listen.

Do not pretend that you heard what someone said when you really didn't. It is not a good idea to pretend. Do not shake your head yes. Do not smile like you understand. The speaker will think you know what was said. This could get you into trouble later. You may be saying yes to something you do not want to do. You may be saying yes without even knowing it!

Why is my health important for speechreading?

It is hard to listen or speechread when you feel sick. Be sure to get enough sleep at night. You do not listen or speechread as well when you feel tired. Eat foods that are good for your body. It can be hard to listen or speechread when you are hungry.

Have your hearing tested every year or two. A hearing test will show if your hearing has changed. It will show if you need a new hearing aid.

Your eyes are just as important as your ears. You cannot speechread without them! Have your eyes tested regularly. This will show if you are seeing well. The doctor will give you glasses if you have trouble seeing. Be sure to wear the glasses if you need them. The glasses will make speechreading easier.

Remember, your health is very important. Take good care of yourself.

How can other people help me to hear better?

Talking to people is easier when they know about your hearing problem. Tell people that you may not hear everything they say. Let them know how they can help you to hear better.

When people are speaking, they can help you in many ways. They will be glad to help you. Let them know when you are having trouble listening or speechreading. Then they can do something to help you. Here is a list of things you can ask people to do.

1. Some people may shout when they talk to you. These people may think you cannot hear them. Ask them not to shout. Tell them your aid makes voices loud enough. Ask them to talk a little slower, not louder.
2. Some people talk very softly. They are hard to hear. Ask them to speak louder.
3. Some people talk too fast. They are hard to understand. Ask them to slow down.
4. Some people always mumble. They are hard to understand. Ask them to speak more clearly.

5. Some people may use long words when they talk. You may not know what the words mean. You may not understand what is being said. Ask people to use words you can understand.
6. You may have trouble hearing when you are away from the person who is talking. The person's voice may sound very soft. Noise may be louder than the voice. You may not hear what is being said. Ask the person to move closer to you. Or, you can move closer to the speaker. You will hear better when you are close to the speaker.
7. Students often have trouble understanding messages given over the loudspeaker in school. You cannot read the speaker's lips because you cannot see the speaker's face. Ask someone to repeat the messages given over the loudspeaker. You can ask a friend or a teacher.
8. It is hard to speechread when you cannot see a speaker's lips. Some people cover their mouths with their hands, a pencil, or a book. Ask them not to put anything in front of their mouths. Tell them you cannot speechread when their faces or mouths are hidden.
9. It is hard to speechread when you cannot see the speaker's face. If the speaker's back is turned to you, ask the speaker to turn around. Ask the speaker to look at you when talking. You must see the speaker's face to speechread.
10. It is hard to speechread when the speaker is standing behind you. You must keep turning around to speechread. Ask the speaker to stand in front of you when talking. Then you will be able to speechread more easily.
11. Some people do not stand still when they talk. They keep moving around. Speechreading is harder when the speaker moves. You can ask people to stand still when they talk. Then you can watch their faces, mouths, and body movements more easily.
12. Many men have a mustache. The mustache may cover a man's lips. Speechreading is harder when the mustache covers the lips. Ask the person to speak a little louder. Stay close to him so that you can hear better.
13. Speechreading is difficult when the speaker is standing in front of a sunny window. The sun will be shining into your eyes. You will have trouble seeing. The speaker's face will be in a shadow. Ask the person to move away from the window.
14. Light is important for speechreading. You cannot speechread unless you can see. Make sure there is enough light in a room for speechreading. Turn on a light if the room is too dark. Then you will see better. You will speechread better.

Lesson 12

What a Hearing Aid Can and Cannot Do

A hearing aid can help you in many ways. But there are some things that it cannot do. An aid cannot do everything for your hearing problem.

Do you understand what a hearing aid can do? Do you understand what it cannot do? Let's see if you do!

EXERCISE 21

Read each sentence. Think about what the sentence says. Put a check under *Yes* if an aid can do what the sentence says. Check under *No* if an aid cannot do what the sentence says.

Check your answers in the Answer Key when you are finished.

A hearing aid:	Yes	No
1. helps me to hear many of the sounds around me.	___	___
2. makes my hearing worse.	___	___
3. helps me to hear better in school.	___	___
4. makes me taller.	___	___
5. helps me even more when I use my eyes with it.	___	___
6. helps me to hear sounds that I could not hear before.	___	___
7. helps me to use the hearing I have.	___	___
8. helps me to tell the difference between noise and important sounds.	___	___
9. cures (takes away) my hearing loss.	___	___
10. makes me hear the same as everyone else hears.	___	___

	Yes	No
11. takes time to get used to.	____	____
12. changes sounds as they go through the aid.	____	____
13. helps me to hear my own voice.	____	____
14. helps me to use better speech sounds when I talk.	____	____
15. helps me to hear while I am sleeping.	____	____
16. helps me the most when I am close to the speaker.	____	____
17. helps me the most when it is quiet.	____	____
18. makes all sounds louder.	____	____
19. makes noises louder.	____	____
20. helps me to hear softer sounds and speech.	____	____
21. makes only speech sounds louder.	____	____
22. makes speech clearer.	____	____
23. helps me to understand speech better.	____	____
24. helps me to hear what other people are saying.	____	____
25. means I do not have to speechread anymore.	____	____

Lesson 13

When Could You Have Trouble Hearing?

There are times when you won't hear what someone says. That's because many things can make listening hard to do. Many things can make speechreading hard to do. These things can keep you from understanding the speaker's words.

When could you have trouble hearing someone? Let's see if you know!

EXERCISE 22

Read each sentence. Think about what the sentence says. Put a check under *Yes* if it could make listening or speechreading hard to do. Check under *No* if it does not make listening or speechreading harder to do.

Check your answers in the Answer Key when you are finished.

It can be hard to understand a speaker when:	Yes	No
1. the speaker talks too fast.	___	___
2. my hearing aid is broken.	___	___
3. the speaker is far away from me.	___	___
4. it is very quiet.	___	___
5. many people are talking at the same time.	___	___
6. I feel tired or hungry.	___	___
7. the speaker talks softly or mumbles.	___	___
8. the speaker stands behind me.	___	___
9. I cannot see the speaker's face or mouth.	___	___
10. the volume on my hearing aid is too low.	___	___

		Yes	No
11.	the speaker looks at me while talking.	___	___
12.	I am not feeling well.	___	___
13.	the room is dark.	___	___
14.	the sun shines in my eyes.	___	___
15.	the speaker has a mustache.	___	___
16.	the speaker stands still while talking.	___	___
17.	the speaker stands in front of a sunny window.	___	___
18.	noise is louder than the speaker's voice.	___	___
19.	a book is in front of the speaker's mouth.	___	___
20.	I wear my hearing aid.	___	___
21.	the speaker talks over a loudspeaker.	___	___
22.	the speaker uses words I do not know.	___	___
23.	some words look the same on the lips.	___	___
24.	the speaker has short hair.	___	___
25.	I am looking out the window instead of watching the speaker.	___	___

Lesson 14

What Can You Do to Hear Better?

There are things you can do to help yourself hear better. You can do things to make listening easier. You can do things to make speechreading easier. These things can help you to understand a speaker's words.

What can you do to hear someone better? Let's see if you know!

EXERCISE 23

Read each sentence. Think about what the sentence says. Put a check under *Yes* if it could make listening or speechreading easier to do. Check under *No* if it does not make listening or speechreading easier to do.

Check your answers in the Answer Key when you are finished.

I can understand a speaker better when I:	Yes	No
1. wear my hearing aid.	___	___
2. make sure my aid is working well.	___	___
3. change my seat.	___	___
4. use my eyes with my hearing.	___	___
5. look at the floor while the speaker talks.	___	___
6. sit up front.	___	___
7. ask the speaker to repeat what was said if I didn't hear it.	___	___
8. wear my glasses (if I have glasses).	___	___
9. get enough sleep at night so I'm not tired.	___	___
10. ask someone to repeat any messages given over the loudspeaker.	___	___

	Yes	No

11. ask a friend to make sure I know about assignments, test dates, or important terms in class.   _____   _____

12. daydream while the speaker is talking.   _____   _____

13. watch the speaker's face, lips, and body movements.   _____   _____

14. move away from things that make noise.   _____   _____

15. ask the speaker to speak loudly and clearly.   _____   _____

16. block out noisy sounds.   _____   _____

17. stay close to the speaker.   _____   _____

18. try to get the general idea of what is being said.   _____   _____

19. worry about words that I missed.   _____   _____

20. can see the speaker's face clearly.   _____   _____

21. pretend I heard what was said.   _____   _____

22. ask the speaker to move away from a sunny window.   _____   _____

23. ask the speaker to stand still while talking.   _____   _____

24. ask the speaker to use words I can understand.   _____   _____

25. turn on a light if the room is too dark.   _____   _____

Lesson 15

How Do You Feel About Your Hearing Aid?

Many people wear a hearing aid. Do you know anyone else who wears an aid? If you do not, you may feel alone. Maybe you would like to talk to someone about how it feels to wear a hearing aid. Talking about your aid can help you to feel better about it. You can talk to your teacher, your parents, or a friend about your hearing aid.

There are many questions about your hearing aid in this section. The answers to these questions are important. The answers will show how you feel about wearing a hearing aid.

After you answer the questions, you will read more about feelings. You will learn some ways to feel better about your hearing aid.

Be honest when you answer these questions. Be honest about your feelings. Do not worry about giving the right answer. There are no right answers or wrong answers. Each person will have different answers.

EXERCISE 24

Read each question. Put a check in front of the best answer. You may have to write a sentence to answer some questions. Everyone will have different answers to these questions. The answers are not in the Answer Key. Show your answers to your teacher.

1. How do you feel about wearing a hearing aid?

    a. _____ I really like to wear it.

    b. _____ I don't mind wearing it.

    c. _____ I don't like to wear it.

    d. _____ Other: _____

2. Do you ever wish that you didn't have to wear an aid?

    a. _____ yes   b. _____ no

3. Do you want to wear an aid so that you can hear better?

   a. _____ yes   b. _____ no

4. Do you think you need a hearing aid?

   a. _____ yes (When/why? _____)

   b. _____ no (Why not? _____)

5. Did you like the aid when you first got it?

   a. _____ yes

   b. _____ no (Why not? _____)

6. What things do you like about your hearing aid? List them.

7. What things don't you like about your hearing aid? List them.

8. How long did it take you to get used to wearing the aid?

9. How does the aid feel while you are wearing it?

   a. _____ It feels good; I hardly know it's there.

   b. _____ It feels all right.

   c. _____ It makes my ear feel full.

   d. _____ It hurts. (Where? _____)

   e. _____ It bothers me. (How? _____)

10. How does the aid sound?

    a. _____ It sounds good.

    b. _____ It sounds bad.

    c. _____ It sounds too soft.

    d. _____ It sounds too loud.

    e. _____ The sounds confuse me.

    f. _____ The sounds give me a headache.

11. An aid makes noise louder. Does the noise ever bother you?

    a. _____ yes (When? _____)

    b. _____ no

12. Can you block out the noises that you hear?

    a. _____ yes   b. _____ no   c. _____ sometimes

13. Does the aid help you hear your own voice better?

    a. _____ yes   b. _____ no

14. Does the aid help you to understand what other people are saying?

    a. _____ yes   b. _____ no

15. Does the aid help you to hear better when you are in a group of people?

    a. _____ yes   b. _____ no

16. Do you use your eyes with your hearing aid?

    a. _____ yes   b. _____ no   c. _____ sometimes

17. Are there any times when the aid does not help you?

    a. _____ yes (When? _____)

    b. _____ no

18. How often do you wear the aid at home?

    a. _____ All the time

    b. _____ Sometimes (When? _____)

    c. _____ Never (Why not? _____)

19. How do you think your parents feel about the hearing aid?

    a. _____ They want me to wear it.

    b. _____ They don't care if I wear it or not.

    c. _____ They don't want me to wear it.

    d. _____ Other: _____

20. Do you have any brothers and sisters? If so, how do you think they feel about the aid?

    a. _____ They want me to wear it.

    b. _____ They don't care if I wear it or not.

    c. _____ They don't want me to wear it.

    d. _____ They make fun of it.

    e. _____ Other: _____

21. Pretend someone asked you, "Is that a hearing aid you are wearing?" How would you feel?

    a. _____ I would not mind it.

    b. _____ I would feel angry about it.

c. _____ I would feel embarrassed.

d. _____ I would feel hurt or sad.

e. _____ Other: _____

22. Pretend someone asked you, "Is that a hearing aid you are wearing?" What would you say?

   a. _____ I would say, "Yes, I wear a hearing aid."

   b. _____ I would say, "No, it's not a hearing aid."

   c. _____ I would say, "It is none of your business!"

   d. _____ I would not answer. I would change the subject and start talking about something else.

23. Do you ever tell anyone that you wear a hearing aid?

   a. _____ yes (Who? _____)

   b. _____ no (Why not? _____)

24. How do you feel about people seeing your hearing aid?

   a. _____ I don't mind if people see it.

   b. _____ I don't want people to see it.

25. How often do you wear the aid when you go to places (for example, to eat out, shop, visit friends, go to parties, or go to the movies)?

   a. _____ All the time

   b. _____ Sometimes (When? _____)

   c. _____ Never (Why not? _____)

26. Do you stay away from people so that they won't see your aid?

   a. _____ yes (Who/when? _____)

   b. _____ no

27. Are you ever afraid people will ask questions about the aid?

   a. _____ yes

   b. _____ no

28. Pretend someone teased you about the hearing aid. How would you feel?

   a. _____ I would not let it bother me.

   b. _____ I would feel angry about it.

   c. _____ I would feel hurt or sad.

   d. _____ Other: _____

29. Pretend someone teased you about the hearing aid. What would you do?

   a. _____ I would ignore it (do nothing).

   b. _____ I would fight back.

   c. _____ I would remove the aid.

   d. _____ I would start to cry.

   e. _____ Other: _____

30. Does wearing an aid make you feel different from other people?

   a. _____ yes (How/when? _____)

   b. _____ no

31. Do you think people ever treat you differently just because you wear a hearing aid?

   a. _____ yes (How/when? _____)

   b. _____ no

32. Do you think you have fewer friends because you wear an aid?

   a. _____ yes (Why? _____)

   b. _____ no

33. Do you know anyone else who wears a hearing aid?

   a. _____ yes (Who? _____)
   (Do you ever talk to them about it? _____)

   b. _____ no

34. Does the aid make you feel more confident in yourself (able to do more things)?

   a. _____ yes (When? _____)

   b. _____ no

35. Does an aid ever stop you from doing something that you would like to do?

   a. _____ yes (What? _____)

   b. _____ no

How to Feel Better About a Hearing Aid

Many people wear hearing aids. You are one of them. You have certain feelings about wearing an aid.

It is helpful to have good feelings about your aid. Good feelings make the aid easier to wear. How can you learn to feel better about your aid? Remember these things.

1. You are not alone! Many people wear a hearing aid.
2. There is nothing wrong with wearing a hearing aid.
3. Tell yourself, "I need an aid to hear better. It is all right to wear an aid."
4. Wearing an aid is easier if you want to wear it. You must want to hear better.
5. Nobody is perfect! Some people need crutches or a wheelchair to move around. Some people wear glasses or braces. You just happen to wear a hearing aid.
6. Don't be afraid to let other people see your hearing aid. If people ask questions about the aid, it means they want to know more about it. Answer all of their questions. Show the aid to them. Explain how it works. Let people listen to the hearing aid.
7. Talking to other people is easier when they know that you wear a hearing aid.
8. An aid does not cause you to have fewer friends. It does not keep you from making friends. Make friends by being friendly to others first. Be cheerful. Say nice things to people. Listen to people when they talk to you. Help others whenever you can. People will be your friend because they like you. They will like you for the way you act. It won't matter to them that you wear a hearing aid.

9. A true friend does not care if you wear a hearing aid.
10. Try to ignore people who make fun of your hearing aid. Some people enjoy teasing others. They do this for attention. They do not care about hurting other people's feelings. They hope you will feel angry or hurt. Don't pay attention to people when they tease you. Then they will stop teasing you. They will stop because you won't be acting the way they want you to. They will not have fun teasing you anymore.
11. Your parents love you very much. They love you even though you wear a hearing aid. It does not matter to them that you wear an aid.
12. It takes time to get used to an aid. Wearing an aid takes much practice. Be patient. Do not give up quickly. Give the aid a fair try. Even if it doesn't seem to help at first, try it again and again.
13. Do not use the aid to get out of doing things. You can do just about everything that other people do, even while wearing the aid.
14. Know how a hearing aid can help you. Know what the aid cannot do for your hearing problem.
15. Know when you may have trouble hearing, even while wearing the aid. Know what things you can do to hear better.
16. You will have mixed feelings about your hearing aid. Sometimes you may feel angry, embarrassed, or sad about wearing an aid. Sometimes you may not like the aid. Don't worry about having these feelings. It is natural to feel all of them. These feelings will last for only a short time. Then they will go away and you will feel better.

Lesson 16

Hearing Aid Care

New Vocabulary

You will learn these words as you read this lesson. Say each word. Read its definition.

Air bulb: a small tool that blows air. It blows out water from inside the hook, tube, and earmold.

Battery tester: a tool that tells how strong a battery is.

Crochet hook: a tool used to crochet. It has a small hook on one end. It can clean wax from the earmold opening.

Damp cloth: a cloth that has a little bit of water on it.

Silica gel: dries out water or sweat from inside a hearing aid.

Wax remover: a tool with a wire loop on one end. It cleans wax from the opening of an earmold.

Taking Care of Your Aid

A hearing aid helps you to hear better when it is working well. You must take good care of the aid for it to work well. The aid will last longer if you take good care of it.

Do you take good care of your hearing aid? Read on to find out!

When You Should Not Wear Your Hearing Aid

There are some times when you should not wear your hearing aid. Do not wear the aid when

1. *you are sleeping:* The aid may hurt your ear when you lie on it. The aid may break if you lie on it.
2. *you take a bath or shower:* The aid won't work well if water gets inside.
3. *you go swimming:* The aid will get wet. Then it won't work well. Also, the aid may get lost in the swimming pool.

4. *you play rough:* The aid can fall off your ear. The aid can get lost or broken while you are playing rough.
5. *you use a hair dryer:* Heat from the hair dryer may hurt the hearing aid.
6. *you put on hair spray:* Hairspray is sticky. It will clog the microphone and make the aid dirty.
7. *you are outside in the rain or snow:* Rain or snow can make the hearing aid wet. Then the aid may not work well.
8. *you are sick:* The aid may not feel good on your ear. If you are lying down, the aid may hurt your ear when you lie on it. The aid may break if you lie on it.
9. *you have a sore ear or when your ear is draining:* The aid may not feel good on your ear.

Put the aid in its own box when you are not wearing it. The box will keep the aid clean. It will keep the aid from getting broken. Put the box in a safe place, like a drawer. A drawer in your bedroom dresser is a good place. Do not put the aid on top of a table or a refrigerator. The aid can fall off and break.

Keep a box for your aid at school. Ask your mother for a small box to keep in school. She may have one in her sewing basket. She may have a small box from a necklace or a ring. Put your aid in the box when you take it off for recess or gym class. Put the box inside your desk or give it to your teacher. Do not leave the aid on top of your desk. It can fall off and break. Do not put the aid inside a book. It can fall out and break, or it can get crushed and break inside the book.

Do not put your hearing aid inside a bookbag along with other books. Books can be very heavy. They can crush the hearing aid. The aid may fall out of the bookbag and get lost or broken.

Never put the aid in your pocket when you are not wearing it. The aid may fall out and break. You may sit on the aid and break it if it is in a back pocket. You may forget to take the aid out of your pocket later. Then it may go into the washing machine when your clothes are washed.

Things That Can Hurt Your Hearing Aid

You must learn to be careful with your hearing aid. Several things can hurt your hearing aid. They are listed here.

1. *Pets:* Dogs and cats can chew on the aid and break it. Keep the aid someplace where they cannot reach it.
2. *Young children:* They may play with the aid and break it. Your hearing aid is not a toy! Teach your younger brothers and sisters not to play with it. Keep the aid someplace where they cannot reach it.
3. *Dropping the aid:* This can break the tiny parts inside the aid. Try not to drop the aid. Do not hit it against anything that is hard. Fix or clean your aid over a table so that it will not fall on the floor. It is helpful to spread a towel over the table. This makes the table top softer in case the aid falls onto the table.

4. *Dirt and dust:* The aid will not work well if dirt and dust get inside. Keep your aid clean. Put the aid in its own box when you are not wearing it. Do not put the aid in your lunchbox. Food and crumbs will make the aid dirty.
5. *Water:* The aid will not work well if water gets inside. Keep your hearing aid dry! Do not set the aid on a sink. Water may splash on it. Do not wear the aid while you are swimming. Do not wear the aid while you are bathing.
6. *Sweat:* Sweat is like water. The aid will not work well if too much sweat gets inside it. Your ears can sweat. Keep your aid dry.
7. *Rain and snow:* Rain and snow are made up of water. Do not let rain or snow touch your aid. Keep the aid covered if you are outside in bad weather.
8. *Heat:* Very hot temperatures can melt a hearing aid. Do not put the aid near anything hot. Do not lay it on a stove or a radiator. Do not wear it while using a hair dryer. Do not wear it while lying under a sun lamp. Do not let it lie in the sun. Do not lay it on a windowsill on a hot, sunny day. Do not leave it in a car that is parked in the sun.
9. *Cold:* Very cold temperatures can make an aid sound weak. The aid will sound weak until it has warmed up. Do not lay the aid in front of an air conditioner. Do not lay it on a cold windowsill. Do not wear the aid outside when the temperature is below freezing.
10. *Toothpicks:* Some toothpicks are very thin. They break easily. Do not use toothpicks to clean your hearing aid. They can break inside the earmold or the tube.
11. *Pipe cleaners and pins:* Pins are sharp. Pipe cleaners can be sharp, too. Do not use them to clean your aid. They can tear a tube or an earmold. They can break a receiver, too.
12. *Hairspray:* Hairspray is very sticky. It makes a hearing aid dirty. It can clog the microphone. Do not spray your hair while you are wearing the aid.
13. *A leaking battery:* A battery can get a hole in it. Water from inside the battery leaks out. It makes the inside of the aid wet. The water dries and makes a hard, white powder. An aid may not work well if a battery leaks inside the case.

Things That Help You Take Care of Your Hearing Aid

Several things will help you take care of your hearing aid. You can find some of these things around your house. You must buy some of them from a store. You must buy some of them from your hearing aid dealer, audiologist, or audiology clinic.

Keep these things together. Put them in a small box, like a shoebox. Then they will be easy to find when you need them.

Here are the things that help you to care for your hearing aid.

1. Always have **extra batteries** at home and at school. Then you will have a strong battery when the old one dies.

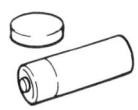

2. Always have **extra cords** at home and at school. Then you will have another cord when the old one breaks.

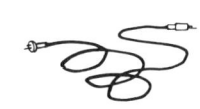

3. Keep a **bar of soap** in the box. Use the soap with warm water. Warm soapy water helps you to wash the earmold, hook, tube, and jacket.

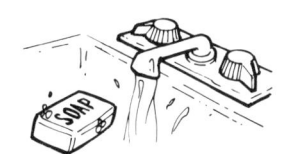

4. Keep a small cloth in the box. When you clean your aid, dampen the cloth. A **damp cloth** has a little bit of water on it. It is not dripping wet! Use a damp cloth to wipe off many parts of your hearing aid.

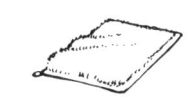

5. A **toothbrush** makes cleaning easier. A dry toothbrush brushes away dirt and dust from the controls of the microphone. Use a toothbrush with soap and water to brush away wax from the earmold.

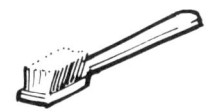

6. A **tiny screwdriver** tightens loose screws in the hearing aid case. Buy a tiny screwdriver from any store.

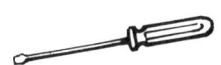

7. A **battery tester** shows how strong a battery is. You can buy a tester for large batteries from your hearing aid dealer, audiologist, or audiology clinic. You can buy a tester for small batteries from a drug store.

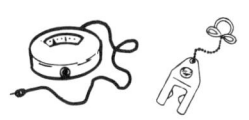

8. A **wax remover** cleans wax from the earmold opening. A wax remover comes with many hearing aids. Did you get one with your aid? If not, buy a wax remover from your hearing aid dealer, audiologist, or audiology clinic.

9. You can use a **crochet hook** to clean the earmold opening. A crochet hook has a small hook on one end. Buy a crochet hook from any store. Maybe your mother has one in her sewing basket. Ask her if you can have it for cleaning your aid.

10. An **air bulb** blows air. It blows out water from inside an earmold or a tube. Buy an air bulb from a hearing aid dealer, audiologist, or audiology clinic.

11. **Silica gel** dries out water or sweat that gets into the hearing aid case. It dries out water or sweat that gets into a receiver, too. Buy silica gel from a hearing aid dealer, audiologist, or audiology clinic.

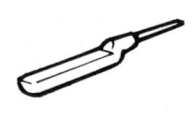

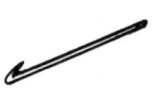

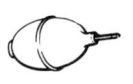

Take your hearing aid to your dealer, audiologist, or clinic once a year. This is very important. They will check your hearing aid. They will do several things.
1. They will put the aid in a special machine. The machine tests the aid. It shows how well the aid is working. It tells if the aid needs to be fixed.
2. They will fix the aid if something is wrong with it.
3. They will put new parts on the aid if it needs any new parts.
4. They will clean the aid on the inside where you cannot reach.
5. They will check your earmold to see if it fits well. If the earmold is too loose, they will make a new one for you.

EXERCISE 25

You have read much about taking care of a hearing aid. Can you answer these questions? Check your answers with the Answer Key when you are finished.

1. When shouldn't you wear a hearing aid? Put a check in front of each correct answer. Find nine answers.

    I should not wear my hearing aid when I:

    a. ____ am sleeping
    b. ____ am in school
    c. ____ am swimming
    d. ____ am sick
    e. ____ take a walk
    f. ____ play rough
    g. ____ watch TV
    h. ____ talk to other people
    i. ____ use a hair dryer
    j. ____ am outside in the rain
    k. ____ take a bath
    l. ____ use hair spray
    m. ____ go to the store
    n. ____ have a sore ear

2. Where is a good place to put your aid when you are not wearing it? Put a check in front of each correct answer. Find four answers.

    When I don't wear my aid, I put it:

    a. ____ in my back pocket
    b. ____ in its own box
    c. ____ on a sink
    d. ____ in a dresser drawer
    e. ____ inside a book
    f. ____ on top of my desk
    g. ____ on a windowsill
    h. ____ where my cat can reach it
    i. ____ in a bag with silica gel
    j. ____ in my lunchbox
    k. ____ on top of a refrigerator
    l. ____ in the teacher's desk

3. Which of these things can hurt your hearing aid? Put a check in front of each correct answer. Find 16 answers.

   a. _____ pets
   b. _____ a clean earmold
   c. _____ a leaking battery
   d. _____ silica gel
   e. _____ hair spray
   f. _____ water
   g. _____ young children
   h. _____ a wax remover
   i. _____ rain or snow
   j. _____ pins
   k. _____ a hair dryer
   l. _____ a soft cloth
   m. _____ a battery tester
   n. _____ dirt and dust
   o. _____ very hot temperatures
   p. _____ very cold temperatures
   q. _____ turning the head very quickly
   r. _____ sweat
   s. _____ toothpicks
   t. _____ pipe cleaners
   u. _____ moving the volume control
   v. _____ dropping the aid
   w. _____ a toothbrush
   x. _____ leaving it in a hot car

4. Write the letter of the correct answer in each blank.

   A. Tiny screwdriver
   B. Silica gel
   C. A dry toothbrush
   D. A wet toothbrush
   E. Extra batteries
   F. Battery tester
   G. Wax remover or crochet hook
   H. Damp cloth
   I. Warm, soapy water
   J. Extra cords
   K. Air bulb

   a. _____ tells how strong a battery is
   b. _____ blows out water from inside an earmold or a tube
   c. _____ washes the earmold, tube, and jacket
   d. _____ used when an old cord breaks
   e. _____ cleans wax from the earmold opening
   f. _____ tightens loose screws in the case
   g. _____ brushes away wax from the earmold with soap and water
   h. _____ wipes off dirt from many parts of a hearing aid

i. _____ used when an old battery dies

   j. _____ dries out water or sweat from inside the case or receiver

   k. _____ brushes away dirt and dust from the microphone or controls

5. How often should you have your hearing aid checked by a hearing aid dealer or audiologist?

   a. _____ once a week

   b. _____ once a month

   c. _____ once a year

Everyone will have different answers to the following questions. The answers are not in the Answer Key. Show your answers to your teacher.

6. Where do you keep your hearing aid when you are not wearing it at home?

   Is it a safe place?   a. _____ yes   b. _____ no

7. Where do you keep your hearing aid when you are not wearing it at school?

   Is it a safe place?   a. _____ yes   b. _____ no

8. Which things do you have at home for taking care of your aid? Put a check in front of each answer. If you do not have all of these things, get them! You need them to take care of your aid.

   a. _____ extra batteries   g. _____ a crochet hook

   b. _____ extra cords   h. _____ a wax remover

   c. _____ a battery tester   i. _____ an air bulb

   d. _____ a soft cloth   j. _____ silica gel

   e. _____ a toothbrush   k. _____ a bar of soap

   f. _____ a tiny screwdriver

9. Do you keep all of these things in one place, like a shoebox or a bag?

   a. _____ yes (Where? _____)

   b. _____ no (You should! Get something to put them in.)

10. Do your ears or your body sweat a lot?

    a. _____ yes (Use silica gel to dry out the sweat.)

    b. _____ no

11. Do you use silica gel?

    a. _____ yes (How often? _____)

    b. _____ no (You should! Buy some silica gel and use it.)

12. When was the last time your aid was checked by a hearing aid dealer or audiologist? Give the date. (Ask your parents if you do not remember.)

13. How old is your hearing aid? (Ask your parents if you do not remember.)

14. In what kind of condition is your hearing aid (how does your aid look)?

    a. _____ good   b. _____ fair   c. _____ poor

Lesson 17

Hearing Aid Parts

Now you will read about the different parts of a hearing aid. You will read about taking care of each part. Your hearing aid will not have all of these parts. Do not read about the parts that your aid does not have.

The Battery and Battery Holder

A battery can die at any time. This is why you should have extra batteries at home. When you buy batteries, buy enough to last for one month. Then you will have batteries when you need them.

Most batteries last about one week. How long your battery lasts depends on how often you wear the aid and how loud you turn the volume control. A battery does not last as long when you wear the aid all the time. This is because the battery is being used more often. A battery dies quicker if you always wear the volume control turned up high. The louder the volume, the more power the battery must use.

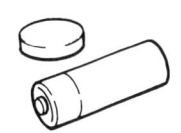

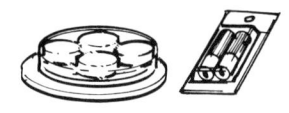

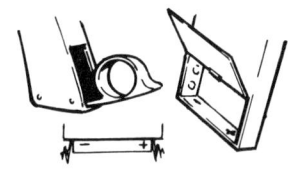

The battery can die while you are in school. Keep one or two batteries in school. Then you can change the battery right away. You will not miss what is said during any classes.

Carry an extra battery with you when you go someplace. A battery may die while you are shopping or visiting someone. It can die while you are seeing a movie or eating in a restaurant. You can change the battery right away if you have an extra one. Then you will not miss what anyone says. You will not miss important sounds, like car horns or sirens.

Keep extra batteries in a cool, dry place. Keep them away from bright light and heat. A closet is a good place to keep extra batteries. A drawer in your bedroom dresser is a good place, too.

Leave the batteries in their own package until you need them. Do not carry batteries loosely in your pocket or purse. If you do, the batteries may touch each other. They may touch other metal objects like keys, pens, or money. This drains the power from a battery. The battery may go dead. It may be dead before you get to use it.

Testing the Battery

A hearing aid will not work with a dead battery. A weak battery can make an aid sound weak or scratchy. The aid may buzz. It may go off and on. Test your battery each morning before putting on the aid. Test it again when you take off the aid. Use only strong batteries in your hearing aid.

A battery tester shows how strong a battery is. Use it to test your batteries. You can buy a tester for large batteries from your hearing aid dealer, audiologist, or audiology clinic. Lay the battery on the tester. Touch it with the wire. The tester will point to a number. The number shows how strong the battery is. You can buy a tester for small batteries from a drugstore. Put the battery inside the tester. The tester will light up if the battery is strong.

There is another way to test your battery. You can test the battery without a battery tester. Hold the hearing aid in your hand. Turn the aid on. Turn the volume control all the way up. Hold the earmold or the receiver next to the microphone. The aid will whistle if the battery is strong. A bone receiver will move if the battery is strong. Put your finger on the bone receiver. You will feel it move.

Taking Care of the Battery

Always buy the right kind of batteries for your aid. The wrong battery can make the aid sound weak or dead. It can make the aid whistle or buzz.

A battery must be put in the aid the right way. Put the " + " on the battery next to the " + " on the hearing aid. An upside-down battery can make the aid sound weak, dead, or scratchy. It can make the aid buzz.

A battery must be clean for the aid to sound right. A battery can get dirty just from touching it with your fingers. Clean the battery if your aid buzzes or sounds scratchy. Wipe the battery with a damp cloth.

A battery can get a hole in it. This makes the battery leak. Water from inside the battery leaks out. Then the battery is no good. A leaking battery can make an aid sound weak or dead. The aid may buzz. It may go off and on.

Do not put a leaking battery into your hearing aid. Throw the battery away. Get a new one. A dead battery can leak. Take a dead battery out of your aid right away.

Always take the battery out of your aid at night. Or, open the battery holder so the battery is not inside the case. Then the battery will not leak inside the hearing aid.

Water from a leaking battery can hurt your hearing aid. The water makes a hard, white powder when it dries. The powder can be on the battery. The powder can be on the battery holder. Powder can go inside the case, too. The powder can make the aid sound weak, dead, or scratchy. The aid may whistle or buzz. It may go off and on.

Other things can make a white powder on the battery or battery holder: sweat from your body, water in the air, and a lot of rain or snow. Use a damp cloth to wipe off any powder from the battery. Clean the battery holder with a damp cloth, too.

Very cold temperatures make a battery weak. The battery will be weak until it has warmed up. It can take one hour for a cold battery to warm up. Some people keep their batteries in the refrigerator. The refrigerator helps their batteries to last longer. Do you keep your batteries in the refrigerator? If so, let a battery warm up before using it.

EXERCISE 26

You have read much about taking care of the battery and battery holder. See if you can answer these questions. Check your answers with the Answer Key when you are finished.

1. Where is a good place to keep extra batteries? Put a check in front of each correct answer. Find five answers.

   I should keep the batteries:

   a. _____ in a drawer
   b. _____ in a metal box
   c. _____ in their own package
   d. _____ in a closet
   e. _____ in silica gel
   f. _____ in a cool, dry place
   g. _____ loose in a pocket or purse
   h. _____ loose with other batteries
   i. _____ away from bright light or heat
   j. _____ on top of the refrigerator

2. What should you do when you are not wearing your hearing aid? Put a check in front of each correct answer. Find three answers.

   When I don't wear my aid, I should:

   a. _____ turn it off.
   b. _____ leave it turned on.
   c. _____ turn the volume control all the way up.
   d. _____ turn the volume control all the way down.
   e. _____ leave the battery inside the hearing aid.
   f. _____ take out the battery or open the battery holder.

3. Why should you take the battery out of your aid at night? Find one answer.

   a. _____ The battery may shrink.

   b. _____ The battery may leak.

   c. _____ The battery may turn purple.

4. Some things can cause a hard, white powder on a battery. What are they? Put a check in front of each correct answer. Find three answers.

   a. _____ popcorn   d. _____ a leaking battery

   b. _____ ice cream   e. _____ an upside-down battery

   c. _____ sweat   f. _____ water from the air, rain, or snow

5. How should you clean the battery and battery holder? Find the best answer.

   a. _____ Rub them with silica gel.

   b. _____ Rub them with a damp cloth.

   c. _____ Scrub them with a scrub brush.

   d. _____ Hold them under your mother's vacuum cleaner.

Everyone will have different answers to the following questions. The answers are not in the Answer Key. Show your answers to your teacher.

6. Where do you buy new batteries for your aid? (Ask your parents if you do not know.)

7. How long does a battery usually last in your hearing aid?

8. What do you do with the old, dead batteries?

9. Do you keep extra batteries at home?

   a. _____ yes (Where? _____)

   b. _____ no (You should. Buy some and keep them at home.)

10. Do you keep extra batteries in school?

    a. _____ yes (Where? _____)

    b. _____ no (You should. Take one or two to school tomorrow.)

11. Do you always carry a battery with you when you go somewhere?

    a. _____ yes (Where do you keep it? _____)

    b. _____ no (You should. Start carrying one with you.)

12. Do you have a battery tester at home?

    a. _____ yes   b. _____ no

13. Do you know how to check your battery with a battery tester?

    a. _____ yes (What do you do? _____)

    b. _____ no (You should. Read page 106 again. Ask someone to show you.)

14. Do you know how to check your battery without a battery tester?

    a. _____ yes (What do you do? _____)

    b. _____ no (You should. Read page 106 again. Ask someone to show you.)

15. Test your battery right now. How strong is it?

    a. _____ It is strong. (Good!)

    b. _____ It is weak. (Get a new battery right now.)

    c. _____ It is dead. (Get a new battery right now.)

16. Do you know how to put the battery (or batteries) in your aid?

   a. _____ yes (Good!)

   b. _____ no (You should. Read page 106 again. Ask someone to show you.)

17. Do you change the battery (or batteries) by yourself?

   a. _____ yes (Good!)

   b. _____ no (You should. Who does it for you? _____)

18. Do you take the battery out of your aid at night?

   a. _____ yes (Good!)

   b. _____ no (You should. Start taking it out.)

19. Has one of your batteries ever leaked?

   a. _____ yes   b. _____ no

20. How does your battery look?

   a. _____ clean (Good!)

   b. _____ dirty (Clean it right now.)

21. How does your battery holder look?

   a. _____ It is clean. (Good!)

   b. _____ It is dirty. (Clean it right now.)

   c. _____ It is broken or cracked. (Take it to a hearing aid dealer or audiologist.)

The Earmold

Keep the earmold clean. Wax on the earmold can make the aid whistle. Check the earmold for wax every day. Clean the earmold when you see wax on it. Clean the earmold at least once a week.

Keep the earmold opening clean. Wax can get inside the opening. The wax gets hard. You can clean the earmold opening with a wax remover. A wax remover has a wire loop on one end. The wire loop pulls out wax from the opening. You can use a small crochet hook to clean the opening, too. A crochet hook has a little hook on one end. The hook pulls out wax from the earmold opening.

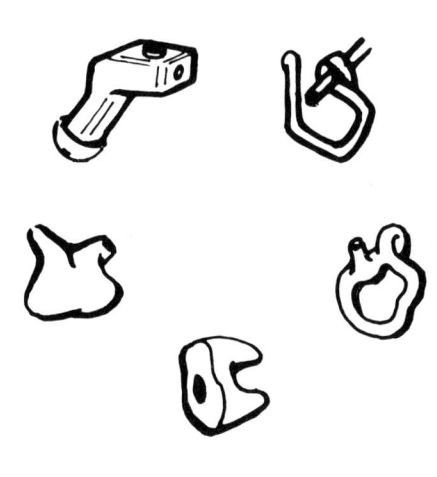

Do not use toothpicks to clean the earmold opening. Toothpicks are thin. They break easily. A toothpick can break inside the earmold. Do not clean the opening with pins or pipe cleaners. They are sharp. They can tear or scratch your earmold.

Wipe a little wax off the earmold with a damp cloth. Wash off heavy wax in warm, soapy water. A wet toothbrush helps to clean the earmold. It brushes away heavy wax very easily. The toothbrush gets into places where your fingers can't.

Do not get the aid wet while washing the earmold. Water can hurt the other parts of your hearing aid. Take the earmold off the aid before washing it.

Some earmolds come apart from the tube. There is a small plastic piece called an **earmold adapter** between the earmold and the tube. The adapter lets you remove the earmold from the tube so you can clean it easily.

Do you have a body aid? If so, take the earmold off the receiver before washing it. Never get the receiver wet!

Do you have a behind-the-ear aid? Take the earmold off the tube if you can. Sometimes the earmold and the tube are one piece. They are glued together. They do not come apart. You must wash the tube with the earmold. Gently pull the tube off the hook. Do not stretch the tube when you pull it off the hook. Hold onto the tube while you are pulling. Do not hold onto the earmold.

Is your hearing aid inside an earmold? If so, never put the earmold into water to clean it! Water will hurt an in-the-ear aid. Wipe the earmold clean with a damp cloth.

An earmold must be dry before you put it back on the aid. It must be dry before you put it into your ear. Wipe the earmold with a dry cloth. Use an air bulb to dry out the opening. An air bulb blows air. It blows out any water from inside the earmold.

Do not blow into the earmold opening with your mouth. This will not dry out the opening. There is water in your mouth. Water from your mouth will go into the earmold. It will make the earmold wet inside.

Having a dry earmold is important. Water from the earmold can go inside the case. This can hurt the hearing aid. Wash your earmold at night. Wash it before you go to bed. Then the earmold will have enough time to dry out. It will be dry before you use it in the morning.

Water or wax can clog the earmold opening. They can stop sound from going into the ear. A clogged earmold can make the aid sound weak or dead. It can make the aid whistle.

The earmold should fit tightly in your ear. A loose earmold can make the aid whistle. Or, the aid may sound weak. Make sure the earmold is all the way in your ear. Make sure it fits well. Your ears grow just as your feet grow. That is why you need a new earmold every one or two years.

A cracked earmold makes an aid whistle. Get a new one from your hearing aid dealer, audiologist, or audiology clinic.

The plastic adapter can wear out from use. After a while, the adapter may not fit tightly to the earmold. That causes the aid to whistle. You must get a new earmold adapter from your hearing aid dealer or audiologist.

Do not wear the aid if there are sores inside your ear. An earmold can make the sores hurt more. Do not wear the aid if your ear is draining. Do not wear the aid if you have an earache.

EXERCISE 27

You have read much about taking care of your earmold. Can you answer these questions? Check your answers with the Answer Key when you are finished.

1. How often should you clean your earmold? Find the best answer.

    a. _____ once a month, even if it is not dirty

    b. _____ when it gets dirty, but at least once a week

    c. _____ only once a year

2. What things could you use to clean the earmold? Put a check in front of each correct answer. Find five answers.

    a. _____ a crochet hook   d. _____ soap and water   g. _____ a dust cloth

    b. _____ a fishing hook   e. _____ a toothbrush   h. _____ a damp cloth

    c. _____ a wax remover   f. _____ a paintbrush

3. Find three things you should not use to clean the earmold. They could hurt your earmold.

    a. _____ a damp cloth   e. _____ a crochet hook

    b. _____ a pin   f. _____ a toothpick

    c. _____ a pipe cleaner   g. _____ soap and water

    d. _____ a wax remover   h. _____ a toothbrush

4. What is the best way to dry the earmold opening?

    a. _____ Use an air bulb.

    b. _____ Put the earmold under a light bulb.

    c. _____ Blow into it with your mouth.

    d. _____ Hold a match near the opening.

5. When is the best time to wash your earmold?

    a. _____ in the morning, before putting the aid on

    b. _____ in the evening, before going to bed

    c. _____ during math class

6. What can happen if you put a wet earmold on your aid? Find one answer.

    a. _____ The water can go inside the case.

    b. _____ The water will drip on my shoes.

    c. _____ The water will get very hot.

    d. _____ The earmold will turn purple.

    e. _____ Nothing will happen. It is okay to put a wet earmold on a hearing aid.

7. What can clog the earmold opening so sound cannot get through? Put a check in front of each correct answer. Find three answers.

    a. _____ sugar   d. _____ silica gel

    b. _____ water   e. _____ a toothbrush

    c. _____ a broken toothpick   f. _____ wax

Everyone will have different answers to the following questions. The answers are not in the Answer Key. Show your answers to your teacher.

8. Do you clean your earmold by yourself?

   a. _____ yes

   b. _____ no (You should. Who cleans your earmold? _____)

9. How often do you clean your earmold?

10. How old is your earmold? (Ask your parents if you do not know.)

    Is it more than two years old?

    a. _____ yes (You may need a new one. Have your dealer, audiologist, or clinic check it.)

    b. _____ no

11. How does your earmold look?

    a. _____ It is clean. (Good!)

    b. _____ It is dirty. (Clean it right now.)

    c. _____ It is broken or cracked. (Get a new one from your dealer, audiologist, or clinic.)

The Case

Keep the case clean. Wipe it with a damp cloth when it gets dirty.

Keep the microphone clean. Wipe the microphone with a damp cloth if dirt or food gets on it. A dry toothbrush brushes away dirt and food, too.

Do not use hair spray while wearing the aid. Hair spray is sticky. It will clog the microphone. It will make the hearing aid dirty. Spray your hair first. Then put on your aid.

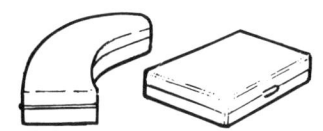

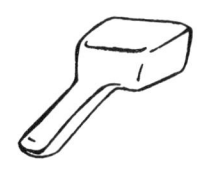

A clean microphone is important. Sound cannot get into a dirty or clogged microphone. The aid will sound weak or dead.

Do not cover the microphone with a hat or a scarf. Do not cover it with heavy clothes. Sound cannot get into the microphone when it is covered. The aid may sound weak. The aid may whistle. The aid will sound scratchy if clothes rub against the microphone.

Do not cover the microphone with your hand. Do not sit where the microphone is too close to a wall. These things can make an aid whistle.

Never get the case wet! Keep the aid covered in bad weather. Water, sweat, rain, or snow can hurt the parts inside the case. A hard, white powder may get on the parts. Then the aid will not work well.

Sometimes the case may get wet. Your aid may fall into a sink or a swimming pool. You may step into the shower while wearing the aid. Rain or snow may get on the aid. Sweat may get inside the case. Don't become scared if the case gets wet. Use silica gel to dry out the case. Put the case in a plastic bag. Put the silica gel in the bag, too. Close the bag tightly. The silica gel will pull out any water from inside the case. Silica gel dries out sweat, too. Use the silica gel before going to bed. The case will be dry when you wake up.

Silica gel does not hurt a hearing aid. It is good for your aid. Use silica gel once a week. Use it even though your aid did not get wet. Silica gel dries out water that you cannot see. It dries out sweat that you cannot see.

Small screws may hold the case together. The screws must be tight. The case can fall apart if the screws are loose. Tighten the screws with a tiny screwdriver.

Never open the case to see what is inside. Never open the case to fix the hearing aid. A hearing aid dealer and an audiologist are the only people who should ever open the case.

See a dealer or audiologist if the case is cracked. See a dealer or audiologist if the aid makes noise when you shake it. Noise means there are loose parts inside the case. A broken case can make the aid sound weak, dead, or scratchy. The aid may whistle or buzz. The aid may go off and on.

EXERCISE 28

You have read much about taking care of the case. Can you answer these questions? Check your answers with the Answer Key when you are finished.

1. Which things can get the case wet? Put a check in front of each correct answer. Find four answers.

    a. _____ water

    b. _____ snow

    c. _____ cake

    d. _____ silica gel

    e. _____ sweat

    f. _____ rain

2. What can happen if the case gets wet? Put a check in front of each correct answer. Find two answers.

    a. _____ The case may get a hard, white powder inside.

    b. _____ The case may crack and break.

    c. _____ The case may shrink.

    d. _____ The hearing aid may not work well.

3. What is the best way to dry out a wet case?

    a. _____ Put it under a sun lamp.

    b. _____ Put it on a stove.

    c. _____ Use silica gel.

    d. _____ Hold a match under the case.

4. How often should you use silica gel? Find the best answer.

   a. _____ only once a year

   b. _____ once a month, even if the case did not get wet

   c. _____ whenever the case gets wet, but at least once a week

5. There are five steps to follow when using silica gel. The steps are listed here. Choose the correct sentence for each step. Put a check in front of each correct sentence.

   Step 1: a. _____ I must get a plastic bag.

   b. _____ I must get a plastic bucket.

   Step 2: c. _____ I must put the hearing aid in the refrigerator.

   d. _____ I must put the hearing aid in the plastic bag.

   Step 3: e. _____ I must put the silica gel under my pillow.

   f. _____ I must put the silica gel in the bag with the aid.

   Step 4: g. _____ I must close the bag tightly.

   h. _____ I must leave the bag open.

   Step 5: i. _____ I must let the silica gel and the aid sit in the bag overnight.

   j. _____ I must let the silica gel and the aid sit in the bag for two hours.

6. What should you use to clean the case? Find one answer.

   a. _____ warm, soapy water

   b. _____ a pencil eraser

   c. _____ a dust cloth

   d. _____ a damp cloth

7. Is it okay for you to open the case of your hearing aid?

   a. _____ yes   b. _____ no

8. Is it okay for your parents to open the case of your aid?

    a. _____ yes   b. _____ no

9. What could you use to clean the microphone? Put a check in front of each correct answer. Find two answers.

    a. _____ a dust cloth   d. _____ toothpaste

    b. _____ a damp cloth   e. _____ a dry toothbrush

    c. _____ a toothpick   f. _____ a wet toothbrush

Everyone will have different answers to the following questions. The answers are not in the Answer Key. Show your answers to your teacher.

10. Do you ever use hair spray?

    a. _____ yes (Do you spray your hair first, then put on the aid? _____)

    b. _____ no

11. Has your case ever gotten wet?

    a. _____ yes (How/when? _____)

    (How did you dry out the case? _____)

    b. _____ no

12. How does your case look?

    a. _____ It is clean. (Good!)

    b. _____ It is dirty. (Clean it right now.)

    c. _____ It is broken or cracked. (Get a new one from your dealer or audiologist.)

13. If your case has screws in it, are they tight?

    a. _____ yes (Good!)

    b. _____ no (Tighten them right now.)

14. How does your microphone look?

    a. ____ It is clean. (Good!)

    b. ____ It is dirty. (Clean it right now.)

    c. ____ It is broken. (Get it fixed by your hearing aid dealer or audiologist.)

The Controls

You should keep the controls clean. They get dirty very easily. They can get dirty just from your fingers. Wipe the controls with a damp cloth to clean them.

Dust may get inside the controls. Dirty or dusty controls can make an aid sound weak. The aid may sound scratchy. The aid may go off and on. Move the controls back and forth a few times to take away some dust. A dry toothbrush brushes away dirt and dust, too.

Always turn the aid off when you are not wearing it. Turn down the volume control. This helps the battery to last longer.

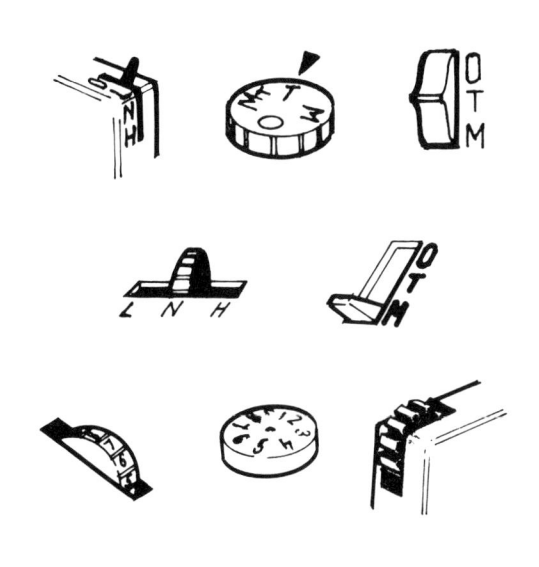

Set the volume control so that it is easy to listen to most sounds. Turn down the volume in noisy places, like the lunchroom or the bus. You can turn up the volume during a class or a spelling test. Do not turn the volume control too high. The aid will whistle if the volume is too high. The aid sounds weak if the volume is too low.

Make sure your aid is set on the right control. For example, when you are in school, you want to hear the teacher. Suppose your aid is not working. What should you do? Check the controls. Is the aid set on *telephone* instead of *microphone*?

Make sure your aid is not set between controls. For example, when you are watching TV, you want to hear the voices. Suppose your aid is buzzing. What should you do? Check the controls. Is the aid set halfway between two letters?

Some hearing aids have a tone control that you can change. The different settings make the aid sound different. The aid must be set on the correct letter. If it is not, the aid won't sound right. The aid may sound weak or different.

The controls should move easily. If the controls break, take your aid to a hearing aid dealer, audiologist, or audiology clinic.

EXERCISE 29

You have read much about taking care of the controls. Let's see if you can answer these questions. Show your answers to your teacher when you are finished.

1. Do you turn the aid off when you are not wearing it?

    a. _____ yes

    b. _____ no (You should! Begin turning it off.)

2. Do you turn down the volume control when you are not wearing the aid?

    a. _____ yes

    b. _____ no (You should! Begin turning it down.)

3. What volume setting do you use for your aid?

    a. _____ very low

    b. _____ halfway between high and low

    c. _____ very high

4. Do you have to turn down the volume in noisy places?

    a. _____ yes (Where? _____)

    b. _____ no

5. Do the controls of your aid move easily?

    a. _____ yes

    b. _____ no (They should! See your hearing aid dealer or audiologist.)

6. Which things should you use to clean the controls? Find two.

    a. _____ a tiny screwdriver

    b. _____ a dry toothbrush

    c. _____ a wet toothbrush

    d. _____ a wax remover

e. _____ floor wax

   f. _____ a damp cloth

7. How do your controls look?

   a. _____ They are clean. (Good!)

   b. _____ They are dirty. (Clean them right now.)

   c. _____ They are broken or cracked. (Get them fixed by your dealer or audiologist.)

The Hook and Tube

A tube can tear very easily. Never twist the tube. Never chew on the hook or tube. A hole in the hook or tube makes an aid whistle.

Keep the hook and tube clean. Wash them in warm, soapy water when they get dirty. Take the hook off the case before washing it. Take the tube off the earmold if you can.

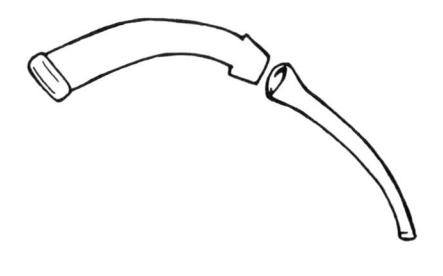

Do not stretch the tube when you pull it off the hook. Gently pull the tube off the hook. An aid sounds different when the tube is stretched.

Sometimes wax gets inside the hook or tube. Use a wax remover to clean out the wax. A wax remover has a wire loop on one end. The wire loop pulls out wax from the hook or tube. A small crochet hook cleans out wax, too. A crochet hook has a little hook on one end. The crochet hook pulls out wax from your hook or tube.

Do not use toothpicks to clean the hook or tube. Toothpicks are thin. They can break inside the hook or tube. Do not use pins or pipe cleaners for pulling out wax. Pins and pipe cleaners are sharp. They can tear a hook or tube. A hole in the hook or tube makes an aid whistle. You must get a new hook or tube from your hearing aid dealer, audiologist, or audiology clinic.

The hook and tube must be dry before you put them on your aid. Use an air bulb to dry them out. An air bulb blows air. It blows out water from inside the hook or tube.

Do not blow into the hook or tube with your mouth. This will not dry them out. There is water in your mouth. Water from your mouth will go into the hook or tube. They will still be wet inside.

Having a dry hook and tube is important. Water from the hook or tube can go inside the case. This can hurt the hearing aid.

Water and wax can clog the hook or tube. Sound cannot get to the earmold when the hook and tube are clogged. The aid may sound weak or dead.

The tube cannot be bent or twisted while you are wearing the aid. Sound cannot get to the earmold. The aid may sound weak or dead.

The tube must fit tightly on the hook. The tube must fit tightly to the earmold. A loose tube can make the aid whistle.

The hook must fit tightly on the case. The aid may whistle if the hook is loose.

A tube is old when it becomes yellow or hard. Most people need a new tube every year. Get a new tube if yours is yellow or hard.

EXERCISE 30

You have read much about taking care of the hook and tube. Can you answer these questions? Check your answers with the Answer Key when you are finished.

1. How should you clean the hook and tube? Put a check in front of each correct answer. Find two answers.

    a. ____ Throw them into the washing machine.

    b. ____ Wash them in warm, soapy water.

    c. ____ Pull a pipe cleaner through them.

    d. ____ Use an air bulb to blow out any wax.

    e. ____ Use a wax remover or a crochet hook.

2. Find three things that you should not use to clean the hook or tube. They could hurt the hook or tube.

    a. ____ a damp cloth

    b. ____ a pin

    c. ____ a pipe cleaner

    d. ____ a wax remover

    e. ____ a crochet hook

    f. ____ a toothpick

    g. ____ soap and water

3. What is the best way to dry out a hook or tube? Find one answer.

   a. _____ Use an air bulb.

   b. _____ Put it under a light bulb.

   c. _____ Blow into it with your mouth.

   d. _____ Hold a hot iron over it.

4. What can happen if you put a wet hook or tube on your aid? Find one answer.

   a. _____ The hook or tube will turn yellow.

   b. _____ The aid will shrink.

   c. _____ The water can go into my eyes.

   d. _____ The water can go inside the case.

   e. _____ Nothing will happen. It is okay to put a wet hook or tube on a hearing aid.

5. Which things can clog a hook or tube so sound cannot get through? Put a check in front of each correct answer. Find three answers.

   a. _____ silica gel

   b. _____ a wax remover

   c. _____ a broken toothpick

   d. _____ water

   e. _____ milk

   f. _____ wax

Everyone will have different answers to the following questions. The answers are not in the Answer Key. Show your answers to your teacher.

6. How often do you clean your hook and tube?

7. Does your hook fit tightly on the case?

   a. ____ yes (Good!)

   b. ____ no (Get a new hook from your dealer, audiologist, or clinic.)

8. How does your hook look?

   a. ____ It is clean. (Good!)

   b. ____ It is dirty. (Clean it right now.)

   c. ____ It has a hole in it. (Get a new hook from your dealer, audiologist, or clinic.)

9. Does your tube fit tightly to the earmold?

   a. ____ yes (Good!)

   b. ____ no (Get a new tube from your dealer, audiologist, or clinic.)

10. Does your tube fit tightly on the hook?

    a. ____ yes (Good!)

    b. ____ no (Get a new tube from your dealer, audiologist, or clinic.)

11. How old is your tube? (Ask your parents if you do not know.)

    Is it more than one year old?

    a. ____ yes (You may need a new one. Have your dealer or audiologist check it.)

    b. ____ no

12. Do you get a new tube every year?

    a. ____ yes (Good!)

    b. ____ no (You should.)

13. Is your tube yellow or hard?

    a. ____ yes (Get a new tube from your dealer, audiologist, or clinic.)

    b. ____ no (Good!)

14. How does your tube look?

   a. ____ It is clean. (Good!)

   b. ____ It is dirty. (Clean it right now.)

   c. ____ It has a hole in it. (Get a new tube from your dealer, audiologist, or clinic.)

The Cord

A cord has many thin wires inside it. These wires can break very easily. That is why an aid needs a new cord more often than any other part. You should have extra cords at home.

The cord may break while you are in school. Keep an extra cord in school. Then you can change the cord right away. You won't miss what is said during any lessons.

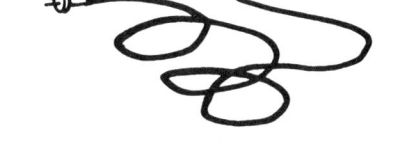

Never chew on the cord. Never tie it into knots. Never twist the cord. These things can break the wires inside the cord.

An aid will not work well if the cord is broken. The aid may sound weak, dead, or scratchy. It may go off and on.

Each cord has a plug on both ends. Hold onto the plug when taking the cord off the aid. Do not pull on the cord! The plugs must fit tightly into the case or the receiver. A loose plug can make the aid sound weak, dead, or scratchy. The aid may whistle or buzz. It may go off and on.

Keep the plugs clean. Wipe them with a damp cloth if they get dirty. Sometimes a white powder gets on the plugs. Water or sweat can cause the white powder to form. Rain or snow can create the white powder, too. Use a damp cloth to wipe off the powder.

White powder or dirt on the plugs keeps the aid from working well. The aid may sound weak, dead, or scratchy. The aid may buzz. If may go off and on.

A cord may look fine on the outside but have broken wires inside. Change the cord if the aid does not work well. Change the cord if a plug is broken.

Always buy the right kind of cord for your aid. The wrong cord makes an aid sound weak or dead.

EXERCISE 31

You have read much about taking care of the cord. See if you can answer these questions. Everyone will have different answers to these questions. The answers are not in the Answer Key. Show your answers to your teacher.

1. Do you keep extra cords at home?

    a. _____ yes (Where? _____)

    b. _____ no (You should. Buy some cords and keep them at home.)

2. Do you keep an extra cord in school?

    a. _____ yes (Where? _____)

    b. _____ no (You should. Take a cord to school tomorrow.)

3. How old is the cord you are now wearing?

    How often do you change the cord on your hearing aid?

4. What do you use to clean the cord and plugs?

5. Does the plug fit tightly into the case of your aid?

    a. _____ yes (Good!)

    b. _____ no (Get a new cord right now.)

6. If your aid has a receiver, does the plug fit tightly into it?

    a. _____ yes (Good!)

    b. _____ no (Get a new cord right now.)

7. How do your plugs look?

    a. ____ They are clean. (Good!)

    b. ____ They are dirty. (Clean the plugs right now.)

    c. ____ They are broken. (Get a new cord right now.)

8. How does your cord look?

    a. ____ It looks good.

    b. ____ It looks broken. (Get a new cord right now.)

    c. ____ It is in knots. (Get a new cord right now.)

The Air and Bone Receivers

Air and bone receivers need the same kind of care. You must keep the receiver clean. Wipe the receiver with a damp cloth when it gets dirty.

Never get the receiver wet! Keep it covered in bad weather. Water, sweat, rain, or snow can hurt the parts inside the receiver. A hard, white powder may get on the parts inside the receiver. Then the aid will not work well. If the receiver gets wet, use silica gel to dry it out. Put the receiver in a plastic bag. Put the silica gel in the bag, too. Close the bag tightly. The silica gel will pull out the water from inside the receiver. Silica gel dries out sweat, too. Use the silica gel before going to bed. The receiver will be dry when you wake up.

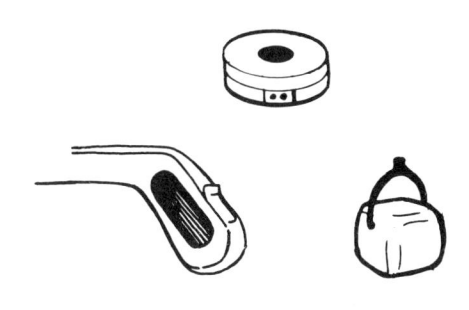

Use silica gel once a week to keep your receiver dry. The silica gel dries out water that you cannot see. It dries out sweat that you cannot see.

An aid whistles when the receiver is too close to the microphone. Move the receiver further away from the microphone. Then the whistling will stop.

An air receiver must fit tightly to the earmold. The aid will whistle if it is loose. See your hearing aid dealer or audiologist if the receiver does not fit tightly to the earmold.

The receiver is a very important part of your hearing aid. Handle it gently. Do not drop the receiver because it can break. A broken receiver can make the aid sound weak or dead. It can make the aid whistle or buzz. The aid may go off and on. Go to a hearing aid dealer, audiologist, or audiology clinic if your receiver is broken.

EXERCISE 32

You have read about taking care of the receiver. Can you answer these questions? Check your answers with the Answer Key when you are finished.

1. What should you use to clean the receiver? Find one answer.

    a. _____ warm, soapy water

    b. _____ a pipe cleaner

    c. _____ a cloth that is damp

    d. _____ a cloth that is dripping wet

2. What can make a receiver wet? Put a check in front of each correct answer. Find four answers.

    a. _____ snow

    b. _____ silica gel

    c. _____ rain

    d. _____ sweat

    e. _____ water

    f. _____ hair spray

3. What can happen if the receiver gets wet? Put a check in front of each correct answer. Find two answers.

    a. _____ The receiver may melt.

    b. _____ The receiver may turn a yellow color.

    c. _____ The receiver may get a hard, white powder inside.

    d. _____ The hearing aid may not work well.

4. What is the best way to dry out a wet receiver? Find one answer.

   a. _____ Use a hair dryer to dry it out.

   b. _____ Use silica gel overnight.

   c. _____ Put it in front of a fan.

   d. _____ Put it in the oven for ten minutes.

5. How often should you use the silica gel? Find the best answer.

   a. _____ only once a year

   b. _____ once a month, even if the receiver did not get wet

   c. _____ whenever the receiver gets wet, but at least once a week

6. How does your receiver look? (Show your answer to your teacher.)

   a. _____ It is clean. (Good!)

   b. _____ It is dirty. (Clean it right now.)

   c. _____ It is broken or cracked. (Get a new one from your dealer, audiologist, or clinic.)

The Jacket and Clip

You should keep the jacket clean. Wash the jacket in warm, soapy water when it gets dirty. Wash it at least once a week. Buy an extra jacket. Then, you will have a jacket to wear while one is being washed.

Do not chew on the jacket. Do not tear it. Sew the jacket if it becomes torn. Buy a new jacket from your hearing aid dealer, audiologist, or audiology clinic.

Many body aids have a clothing clip. The clip holds the aid onto a shirt pocket. Use the clip if you do not want to wear the jacket.

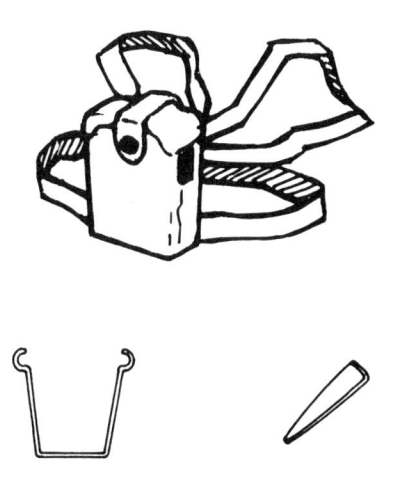

Some clothing clips come off the hearing aid. Put the clip in a safe place when you take it off the aid. A drawer in your bedroom dresser is a good place to put the clip. Then the clip won't get lost.

Wipe the clip with a damp cloth if it gets dirty. Buy a new clip from a dealer, audiologist, or audiology clinic if yours breaks.

EXERCISE 33

Can you answer these questions about taking care of the jacket and clip? Check your answers with the Answer Key when you are finished.

1. How often should you wash the jacket? Find the best answer.

    a. _____ only once a year

    b. _____ whenever the jacket gets dirty, but at least once a week

    c. _____ once a month, even if the jacket is not dirty.

2. How can you clean the jacket? Find two answers.

    a. _____ Brush it with toothpaste and a toothbrush.

    b. _____ Wash it in a mud puddle.

    c. _____ Wash it in a sink.

    d. _____ Put it in the washing machine.

3. What should you use to clean the clip? Find one answer.

    a. _____ a damp cloth

    b. _____ a dirty rag

    c. _____ a washing machine

    d. _____ a pipe cleaner

Everyone will have different answers to the following questions. The answers are not in the Answer Key. Show your answers to your teacher.

4. How often do you use the jacket to hold the aid near your chest?

    a. _____ always   b. _____ sometimes   c. _____ never

5. How often do you wash your jacket?

6. How does your jacket look?

   a. _____ It is clean. (Good!)

   b. _____ It is dirty. (Wash it right now.)

   c. _____ It is torn. (Sew it right now.)

   d. _____ I lost it. (Get a new one from your dealer, audiologist, or clinic.)

7. How often do you use the clip to hold the aid on a shirt pocket?

   a. _____ always   b. _____ sometimes   c. _____ never

8. Does your clip come off the hearing aid?

   a. _____ yes (Where do you put the clip when you take it off? _____)
      (Is that a safe place? _____)

   b. _____ no

9. How does your clip look?

   a. _____ It is clean. (Good!)

   b. _____ It is dirty. (Clean it right now.)

   c. _____ It is broken. (Get a new one from your dealer, audiologist, or clinic.)

   d. _____ I lost it. (Get a new one from your dealer, audiologist, or clinic.)

The Headband and Frames

You must keep the headband or frames clean. Use a damp cloth to clean the headband or frames when they get dirty.

Do not chew on the headband or frames. Do not twist them.

The headband or frames should fit tightly on your head. They must fit tightly to hold the hearing aid close to your ear.

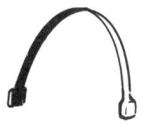

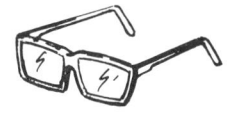

A bone receiver should be tight against the bone behind your ear. A loose bone receiver causes the aid to sound weak or scratchy. Or, the aid may whistle. That is why the headband or frames must be tight.

Bend the headband so the receiver fits over the bone behind your ear. Ask your parents, hearing aid dealer, or audiologist to bend the frames for you.

See your hearing aid dealer or audiologist if the headband or frames break.

EXERCISE 34

Can you answer these questions about taking care of the headband or frames? Everyone will have different answers to these questions. The answers are not in the Answer Key. Show your answers to your teacher.

1. How does your headband or frame fit on your head?

    a. _____ It fits tightly.

    b. _____ It is loose. (Ask your parents, audiologist, or hearing aid dealer to bend it.)

2. How does your headband or frame feel while you are wearing it?

    a. _____ It feels good.

    b. _____ It hurts. (Where? _____)
    (Ask your parents or hearing aid dealer to bend it.)

3. How do you clean your headband or frames?

    a. _____ I rub it with silica gel.

    b. _____ I rub it with a pencil eraser.

    c. _____ I wipe it with a dirty rag.

    d. _____ I wipe it with a damp cloth.

4. How does your headband or frame look?

    a. _____ It is clean. (Good!)

    b. _____ It is dirty. (Clean it right now.)

    c. _____ It is broken or cracked. (Get a new one from your dealer, audiologist, or clinic.)

Lesson 18

Fixing Hearing Aid Problems

A hearing aid has many parts. There can be problems with each part. The aid won't work well when something is wrong with just one part. Your aid has a problem if—
1. it is dead;
2. it sounds weak;
3. it sounds scratchy;
4. it whistles;
5. it buzzes;
6. it goes off and on.

Sometimes your hearing aid may not work well. There may be a problem with it. You must look at the aid to find out what is wrong with it. Try to fix the problem yourself.

There are some hearing aid problems that you cannot fix. If there is a problem inside the aid, you must take the aid to your hearing aid dealer or audiologist. You should never open the hearing aid case yourself. Only hearing aid dealers and audiologists should open the case.

Hearing aid dealers and audiologists can fix many problems in their offices. But there are some problems they cannot fix by themselves. They sometimes send aids to the factory to be fixed. Your hearing aid may be at the factory for several weeks. If this happens, you can borrow an aid from the hearing aid dealer or audiologist.

The following chart lists different hearing aid parts. The list is in alphabetical order. You will see problems that each part can have. You will find out how to fix the problems, too.

Look at the chart when your hearing aid is not working well. Find the parts that belong to your aid. Read about each problem the part can have. Check your aid to see if there is a problem with that part. Read how to fix the problem. The chart will also tell you when you should take the aid to your hearing aid dealer or audiologist to be fixed.

How to Fix Your Hearing Aid

Hearing Aid Part	Problem	Solution
Battery	dead	change the battery
	weak	change the battery
	wrong kind	change the battery
	leaking	change the battery
	dirty	clean battery with a damp cloth
	white powder on battery	clean battery with a damp cloth or change the battery
	upside-down in aid	put battery in aid correctly
	cold	let battery warm up
Battery Holder	dirty	clean holder with a damp cloth
	white powder inside holder	clean holder with a damp cloth
	broken or cracked	take the aid to your dealer or audiologist
Case	water or sweat inside	dry with silica gel
	cold case	let aid warm up
	loose parts inside	take the aid to your dealer or audiologist
	broken or cracked	take the aid to your dealer or audiologist
Controls	dirty or dusty controls	clean with a damp cloth or a dry toothbrush
	volume too low	turn up volume control
	volume too high	turn down volume control

How To Fix Your Hearing Aid (continued)

Hearing Aid Part	Problem	Solution
Controls (continued)	aid turned off	turn microphone on
	aid set on telephone	turn microphone on
	aid set between letters	move control to correct letter
	wrong tone control setting	move control to correct letter
	broken or cracked controls	take the aid to your dealer or audiologist
Cord	wrong kind	change cord
	broken cord	change cord
	broken plug	change cord
	loose plug	push plug firmly into aid
	dirty plugs	clean with a damp cloth
	white powder on plugs	clean with a damp cloth
Earmold	wax on earmold	clean in warm, soapy water
	wax inside opening	clean with a wax remover or a crochet hook
	water inside opening	dry with an air bulb
	not in ear tightly	push earmold firmly into ear
	too small for ear	take the earmold to your dealer or audiologist
	broken or cracked	take the earmold to your dealer or audiologist
	loose fit to earmold adapter	take the aid to your dealer or audiologist

How To Fix Your Hearing Aid (continued)

Hearing Aid Part	Problem	Solution
Hook	wax inside	clean with a wax remover or a crochet hook
	water inside	dry with an air bulb
	hole in hook	take the aid to your dealer or audiologist
	loose fit between hook and case	take the aid to your dealer or audiologist
Microphone	dirty or clogged	clean with a damp cloth or a dry toothbrush
	covered up	uncover microphone
	clothing rubbing against microphone	do not put much clothing over microphone
	microphone too close to receiver	move microphone away from receiver
	microphone too close to a wall, hand, etc.	move microphone away from the object
Receivers		
Air	water or sweat inside	dry with silica gel
	broken or cracked	take the aid to your dealer or audiologist
	loose fit between receiver and earmold	take the aid to your dealer or audiologist
Bone	water or sweat inside	dry with silica gel
	broken or cracked	take the aid to your dealer or audiologist
	loose fit against bone behind the ear	bend the headband or frames for tighter fit against head

How To Fix Your Hearing Aid (continued)

Hearing Aid Part	Problem	Solution
Tube	wax inside	clean with a wax remover or a crochet hook
	water inside	dry with an air bulb
	bent or twisted	straighten tube
	hole in tube	take the aid to your dealer or audiologist
	stretched tube	take the aid to your dealer or audiologist
	loose fit between tube and hook	take the aid to your dealer or audiologist
	loose fit between tube and earmold	take the aid to your dealer or audiologist

EXERCISE 35

You have read much about fixing hearing aid problems. See if you can answer these questions. Check your answers with the Answer Key when you are finished.

1. Only two people should open the case to fix a problem with your hearing aid. Who are they? Find two answers.

   a. _____ I can open the case because it is my hearing aid.

   b. _____ My parents can open the case because they bought the aid.

   c. _____ My audiologist can open the case.

   d. _____ My grandfather can open the case because he is very good at fixing things.

   e. _____ A hearing aid is like a small radio. A person who fixes radios can open the case to fix my aid.

   f. _____ My hearing aid dealer can open the case.

2. Which of these hearing aid problems can you or your parents easily fix? Put a check in front of each correct answer. Find eight answers.

   a. _____ a broken earmold

   b. _____ white powder on the battery

   c. _____ water inside the case

   d. _____ loose parts inside the case

   e. _____ a broken control

   f. _____ a control set between letters

   g. _____ water inside the tube

   h. _____ a broken receiver

   i. _____ a cracked earmold

   j. _____ a broken cord

   k. _____ a torn tube

   l. _____ a clogged earmold

   m. _____ a dirty microphone

   n. _____ a loose plug

3. Have you ever taken your aid to a dealer to be fixed? (Show your answer to your teacher.)

   a. _____ yes (What was the problem? _____)
   (Did you borrow an aid while yours was being fixed? _____)

   b. _____ no

Summary

You have worked very hard on this book. It took a long time to do. You did a good job!

Think about all the things you have learned. You know how our ears work. You know what causes people to have a hearing loss. You understand the different kinds and amounts of hearing loss. You know how hearing is tested for sounds and speech. You understand your audiogram.

You know the different kinds of hearing aids and how they work. You know how and when an aid helps you. You understand what an aid cannot do for you. You know how to take care of your hearing aid. You know how to fix small problems with it.

Congratulations! You have learned a lot. This book will always help you take care of your hearing aid. Put the book in a safe place where you will remember it. Then, you can use it whenever you need it.

Answer Key

EXERCISE 1

1. a. F   f. F
   b. F   g. T
   c. T   h. T
   d. F   i. F
   e. T

2. a. cochlea
   b. eardrum
   c. brain
   d. hearing nerve
   e. hammer, anvil, and stirrup

3. a. pinna   g. cochlea
   b. ear canal   h. nerve endings
   c. eardrum   i. hearing nerve
   d. hammer   j. outer ear
   e. anvil   k. middle ear
   f. stirrup   l. inner ear

EXERCISE 2

1. a. sound wave
   b. decibel
   c. frequency
   d. a jet engine
   e. the *sh* in shoe
   f. no

2. a. waves
   b. second
   c. far apart
   d. lower
   e. hertz

EXERCISE 3

1. A person can have a conductive loss if he or she—
   - has no pinna
   - has a blocked ear canal
   - has no eardrum
   - has a hole in the eardrum
   - has no bones in the middle ear
   - has bones that grew together
   - has fluid in the middle ear
   - was hit on the head very hard

2. A person can have a nerve loss if he or she—
   - was born too early
   - was very sick
   - had a very high fever
   - had a bad reaction to some medicine
   - was hit on the head very hard
   - listened to loud noises or loud music a lot
   - has a relative with a nerve loss
   - grows older and the nerve endings do not respond to sounds

3. a. mixed loss _____ outer, middle, and inner ear
   b. conductive loss _____ outer ear and middle ear
   c. nerve loss _____ inner ear

4. a. T
   b. F
   c. F
   d. T
   e. F

EXERCISE 4

1. a. B
   b. D
   c. C
   d. A

2. a. F
   b. F
   c. T
   d. F

3. b and f

EXERCISE 5

1. a, c, and d
2. b, c, d, f, h, and i
3. a, c, d, g, h, and j
4. a, b, c, e, f, h, i, k, and l

EXERCISE 6

1. a. a person _____ an audiologist
   b. a chart _____ an audiogram
   c. a machine _____ an audiometer
   d. a place _____ an audiology clinic

2. a. T
   b. F
   c. F
   d. T
   e. F

3. c

4. a, b, c, and f

5. a. 20 to 40 decibels _____ a mild hearing loss
   b. 40 to 60 decibels _____ a moderate hearing loss
   c. 60 to 90 decibels _____ a severe hearing loss
   d. 90 to 110 decibels _____ a profound hearing loss

6. a, c, d, and e

7. b, c, and e

8. a. right ear
   b. left ear
   c. left ear
   d. right ear
   e. left ear

EXERCISE 7

1. a, b, d, e, h, i, and k

2. a, e, g, i, j, k, and l

EXERCISE 8, 9, 10, 11, and 12

Show your answers to your teacher.

EXERCISE 13

1. a. S
   b. S, H, O
   c. O
   d. H
   e. S
   f. O
   g. H
   h. H
   i. O
   j. S, H, O
   k. S
   l. S, O
   m. S, H
   n. S, H, O
   o. H
   p. S, O
   q. H, O
   r. O
   s. S, H, O
   t. S, O

2. Show your chart to your teacher each time you fill in a line.

EXERCISE 14

1. a. F
   b. F
   c. F
   d. T
   e. T
   f. F
   g. T
   h. F
   i. T
   j. F

2 and 3. Show your answers to your teacher.

EXERCISE 15 and 16

Show your answers to your teacher.

EXERCISE 17

1. The battery supplies power to make the aid work.
2. The battery holder holds the battery inside the aid. On some aids, the battery holder turns the aid on and off. The aid is turned on when the battery holder is closed; it is turned off when the holder is opened.
3. The case is the outside covering of the aid. It covers the wires and tiny parts inside the aid. The case keeps the wires and tiny parts from getting dirty or lost.
4. The screws hold the case together so the inside parts don't fall out.
5. The microphone pulls sounds, noise, and speech into the hearing aid.
6. The on-off control turns the aid on and off. Every hearing aid is different. Sometimes the battery holder or the volume control turns the aid on and off. Different hearing aids can have different letters printed on them. *O* often means the aid is turned off. *M* often means the microphone is turned on. *S* or *H* often mean the microphone will block out louder, noisy sounds. Your hearing aid may have different letters than these.
7. The volume control makes the aid sound louder or softer. On some aids, the volume control is also the on-off control.
8. The tone control makes some sounds louder than other sounds. *L* means that low sounds are being made louder. *H* means high sounds are being made louder than other sounds. *N* means that no sounds are louder than others. All low, middle, and high sounds have the same loudness.
9. The telephone control helps a person to hear better over the telephone. *T* often means the microphone is picking up sounds from the telephone.
10. The microphone and telephone control makes the microphone control and telephone control work at the same time. *MT* or *B* often means the microphone will pick up sounds from a telephone. It will also pick up sounds from a special set of wires around a room.
11. The hook fits over the ear and holds the aid on the ear. The hook carries sound from the aid to the tube.
12. The tube carries sound from the hook to the earmold.
13. The cord on a body aid is a wire that carries sounds from the case to the receiver. The cord on cross-over aids is a wire that carries sounds from one hearing aid to the other.
14. The earmold fits into the ear. It sends sounds from the hearing aid into the outer ear.
15. An air receiver sends sounds from the hearing aid into the earmold.

16. A bone receiver sends sounds from the aid into the inner ear. The bone receiver moves back and forth behind the ear. It makes the bones of the head move.
17. The clip holds a body aid onto a person's clothes.
18. The jacket is a special pocket that holds a body aid near the chest.
19. A headband goes on the head. It holds a bone receiver on the bone behind the ear.
20. The frames are one part of an eyeglass aid. The frames hold the hearing aid near the ear.

EXERCISE 18

Show your drawing to your teacher.

EXERCISE 19

Show your chart to your teacher each time you fill in a line.

EXERCISE 20

1. b
2. c
3. c
4. a, d, f, and g
5. b and e
6. a and d
7. e
8. Show your answers to your teacher.

EXERCISE 21

1. yes
2. no
3. yes
4. no
5. yes
6. yes
7. yes
8. yes
9. no
10. no
11. yes
12. yes
13. yes
14. yes
15. no
16. yes
17. yes
18. yes
19. yes
20. yes
21. no
22. no
23. yes
24. yes
25. no

EXERCISE 22

1. yes	9. yes	17. yes
2. yes	10. yes	18. yes
3. yes	11. no	19. yes
4. no	12. yes	20. no
5. yes	13. yes	21. yes
6. yes	14. yes	22. yes
7. yes	15. yes	23. yes
8. yes	16. no	24. no
		25. yes

EXERCISE 23

1. yes	9. yes	17. yes
2. yes	10. yes	18. yes
3. yes	11. yes	19. no
4. yes	12. no	20. yes
5. no	13. yes	21. no
6. yes	14. yes	22. yes
7. yes	15. yes	23. yes
8. yes	16. yes	24. yes
		25. yes

EXERCISE 24

Show your answers to your teacher.

EXERCISE 25

1. a, c, d, f, i, j, k, l, and n

2. b, d, i, and l

3. a, c, e, f, g, i, j, k, n, o, p, r, s, t, v, and x

4.
   a. F
   b. K
   c. I
   d. J
   e. G
   f. A
   g. D
   h. H
   i. E
   j. B
   k. C

5. c

6 to 14. Show your answers to your teacher.

EXERCISE 26

1. a, c, d, f, and i

2. a, d, and f

3. b

4. c, d, and f

5. b.

6 to 21. Show your answers to your teacher.

EXERCISE 27

1. b

2. a, c, d, e, and h

3. b, c, and f

4. a

5. b

6. a

7. b, c, and f

8 to 11. Show your answers to your teacher.

EXERCISE 28

1. a, b, e, and f

2. a and d

3. c

4. c

5. a, d, f, g, and i

6. d

7. b

8. b

9. b and e

10 to 14. Show your answers to your teacher.

EXERCISE 29

Show your answers to your teacher.

EXERCISE 30

1. b and e

2. b, c, and f

3. a

4. d

5. c, d, and f

6 to 14. Show your answers to your teacher.

EXERCISE 31

Show your answers to your teacher.

EXERCISE 32

1. c

2. a, c, d, and e

3. c and d

4. b

5. c

6. Show your answer to your teacher.

EXERCISE 33

1. b

2. c and d

3. a

4 to 9. Show your answers to your teacher.

EXERCISE 34

Show your answers to your teacher.

EXERCISE 35

1. c and f

2. b, c, f, g, j, l, m, and n

3. Show your answer to your teacher.